I0416914

Missed Conception

Trying to Conceive with P.C.O.S.

Katherine Shields

Copyright © 2015 Katherine Shields

All rights reserved.

ISBN-13: 978-1502812025

There is no greater agony
than bearing an untold story
inside you.

Maya Angelou

Katherine Shields

But Don't tell Anyone
Prologue

The feminist movement fought to allow women to have freedom and choices without condemnation. Despite this, a woman still can not escape being asked the same two questions: "When are you going to get married?" and "When are you going to have children?" Despite innocent intentions, these questions can easily make a woman feel pretty condemned.

As soon as I was married, if people saw me out to dinner without a glass of wine, I was instantly asked if were pregnant. A woman should be able to choose whether or not to enjoy a little vino without discussing the activities of her uterus.

When I did enjoy a little wine, during the time we were taking breaks from fertility treatments, I inevitably would let it slip to someone that we were doing fertility. The guilt would creep in the next day for fear I had perhaps made them uncomfortable or that they would tell someone who would leak our secret out to everyone. After a year and a half of trying to hold in that we were going through fertility treatments, it began to really take a toll on my soul.

I am the type of person who tells all anyway. There is no filter whatsoever. In the following chapters, you will see how blatantly obvious that is. Keeping a secret that my life decisions, thoughts, prayers and hopes revolve around is agonizing.

Even simple daily tasks like grocery shopping can be torturous. Several times at the grocery store, it seemed every aisle had a cart with a newborn in it. The cries would tear at me, and I would long to have a baby of my own. Babies are everywhere. They are unavoidable.

The anger that wells up in a person who is experiencing frustration and depression is frightening and very powerful. Yes, my hormones were out of control, but the immense anger that I felt over not being pregnant could do the damage of a tsunami.

Having to be around women who were making poor choices during their pregnancies made me want to shake them. Thinking about women who might get pregnant before me was just as devastating. I realize that I am not portraying that I handled infertility gracefully. That is because I didn't.

I could literally feel myself falling apart with bitterness.

The ironic thing is I never stopped believing I would be a mother. I so wanted it to happen like it seemed to happen for everyone else. I just wanted to experience the, "Oh, I think I'm late on my period. I better take a test. Wow, I am pregnant!" I didn't want my husband to ever have to know the details of ovulating or for another man to inseminate me in a fertility office.

I told myself my child would be more anticipated and treasured than most. While I do believe this, it was not enough to bring calmness.

There are always fertility stories out there to make you realize it could be so much worse. What perhaps could make them all a little more bearable is eliminating the infamous, "but don't tell anyone."

"But don't tell anyone" means no sympathy cards or flowers. No pat on the back to say, "You're going to get through this!" or

"How are you feeling today?"

Why is a health diagnosis that plagues 10-15% of the population so rarely discussed? As if the needles, exams, emotions and debt of infertility are not enough, there is also often the pressure to only talk to your partner about the treatments and all the accompanying stressors.

I AM INFERTILE! I CAN'T HAVE A BABY ON MY OWN. THE ONE THING I EVER WANTED IN LIFE MAY NOT HAPPEN AND CERTAINLY WON'T HAPPEN AS EASILY AS IT DOES FOR OTHERS. THERE ARE TIMES WHEN I CAN'T SEE THE BRIGHT SIDE!

Then the anger began to fade. When I began to tell people, support flooded in, and the loneliness of the situation faded out. People learned to stop asking, "When are you having kids?" Every once in a while, someone would engage in the conversation with relief in being able to share their own struggles, and I would be reminded of the *one* other woman I know who spoke openly about her journey in a crowded room to me.

Yes, there were also the people who made ignorant comments. Of course, they hurt. There were far more supportive and encouraging comments though that helped keep me focused on why I was going through this and how sweet the reward would be.

Again, I know that baby or no baby, I have a blessed life. I know other women deserve to have children. I understand that there are more devastating things to go through in life. But until the silence is broken on infertility, people will agonize in solitude instead of be uplifted with hope in the embrace of a supportive community.

I am by no means an expert or a doctor. All statistics, medical suggestions and other health references are simply my understanding. Every journey of infertility is relative. I am one woman with PCOS, and this is *my* story.

Part One

Missed Conception

P.C.O. –What?
Chapter 1

I had my latest T.J. Maxx find of designer sunglasses on my head, and a Diet Coke in the cup holder. I was twenty-one, and on my way to a couple of classes before I headed to work. Those days, I was driving a champagne, Nissan Sentra (everything sounds classier when described as "champagne"), and still listening to that old Alanis Morisette CD.

A car looking for the airport made a quick turn from the center lane and T-boned in to me. The airport was about thirty miles away, but their urgent need to turn that second, landed my car into a telephone pole.

I was sore from hip to hip from the seatbelt, but I assumed that would go away in a few days. In the next couple of months, I gained 20 pounds (weight: 152), and the pain in my hips increased.

I finally went to my doctor who asked if my periods were normal. What did this possibly have to do with the wreck and my weight gain? However, come to think about it, my periods had not been normal since long before the wreck.

So the doctor then prescribed me an ultrasound and sent me to a specialist. She didn't think my symptoms had anything to do with the car accident.

A few weeks later, I followed up with whom would be the first of many specialists. While lying on my back, feet in stirrups, the doctor announced that my uterus looked healthy.

"I have a uterus!" I thought. Does that mean I am pregnant? How could this be? I don't even have a boyfriend right now! Oh, wait, "uterus," I'm thinking "placenta."

Okay, back to focusing on what this woman with the plastic, not-so-magical wand up me is saying. The specialist proceeds to announce she is diagnosing me with something called "Polycystic Ovarian Syndrome. PCOS."

"Syndrome?" That's never good. "Ovarian" something? That's not good either! Of all my body parts, not my girl parts! This could severely derail my plans for my M.R.S. degree.

The small-framed, Asian doctor then digressed from the diagnosis with the declaration, "You too fat." No shit lady, I told you one of the reasons I knew something was wrong was from my weight gain.

The doctor went on to explain that PCOS was an endocrine system disorder. My body now struggled to regulate insulin and sugar which was causing the weight gain. Also, it would now be harder to lose the weight. She wanted me to begin taking the diabetes drug, Metformin, and start to test my blood sugar a couple of times a day.

According to the doctor, this "syndrome" was also the cause of my struggle with ovulation and the lack of regular periods. So a prescription was written for birth control in order to regulate my cycle.

Oh, and the facial hair that I recently had been blessed with? That too was a symptom of PCOS. As far as the facial hair was concerned, the doctor suggested another pill she could prescribe. Then she informed me I would have to have my liver tested frequently to make sure it was not shutting down. I decided to choose to keep a healthy liver and just keep up the waxing.

The doctor then asked, "Have you experienced any depression?"

Well, what do you think? I've become fat, hairy and am in pain. At the moment, the peach fuzz was about the only thing in my life that seemed peachy. But dramatics aside, I was in my early 20's and making the most of parties, friends and the pool. So I decided to pass on the therapy and support groups the doctor had suggested. . . . (Who knew how badly I would need them later!)

After all that had been discussed, the specialist sent me on my way – back to the Sentra, that now had a crooked bumper.

I skipped class that evening and instead went out to dinner with a friend. There are worse things to be diagnosed with. I understand that, but a diagnosis is never a good thing, and dinner with a girlfriend is always a good thing.

The next morning I started the Metformin. I quickly realized that my new unwanted alarm clock would be getting sick at 5:25 on the dot every morning. If only I could have found a snooze button for the side effects.

After the doctor expressed her severe disappointment in me that my body wasn't even tolerating Metformin's medium dosage (as if this was a personal attack against her), I decided I no longer needed to take it. I did stay on the birth control and resolved to believe this problem would not be such a problem.

* * *

A little over a year later, I met the man who would eventually be my husband. A couple months in to dating, my recent diagnosis was weighing on my mind.

I decided that I should come up with some imaginary friends who were in situations of infertility. This may sound a little crazy, but I never said I wasn't. To my credit, I knew from day one we would get married someday. I know it sounds like a cheesy chick flick, except I am by no means a cute, skinny blonde. Also, keep in mind, I had one mission in my early twenties: find a man, marry, and have beautiful babies . . . and be magically, financially stable somehow too.

Anyways, the boyfriend-eventually-turned-husband seemed supportive of people who adopted and also talked about wanting kids someday. This was good enough for the time being.

I don't remember exactly when I had the conversation with my husband (at the time boyfriend) that I had PCOS. It was probably in bits and pieces or I would be able to remember a formal conversation about it. I do know that it was before we got engaged, because I personally would have truly had to reconsider marrying someone if I knew there was a risk that they would not be fertile. That might be shallow, but it is honest. So I knew I owed the full disclosure to him.

I do remember the first time I realized he got the potential severity of the diagnosis. One day I was complaining about my weight, as I often do. He started the typical "Oh, you are beautiful baby." Then he proceeded to say, "but if you are that bothered by it, I read where you should really be avoiding white carbs."

The way he said it, just keyed me in to realizing the "you" was not the general population that should be staying away from white carbs, but specifically "PCOS me." When I mockingly asked him where he read such a revelation, he said he'd been looking up "things" on the internet about PCOS. The fact that my non-studious boyfriend had been researching about my medical condition, made it undeniable that this *was* something that concerned him.

One month my period was especially frustrating. This was during the incredibly long phase of, "is he going to propose or not." He jokingly made a comment about why was I surprised my period was irregular since I had "damaged goods."

Instantly, I assumed this was why the proposal had yet to happen. I can assure you, because of my reaction, that he has never used those words again. While he thought he was being funny, he had uttered my greatest fear.

* * *

We did get engaged (obviously since we are now married), and I began immediately planning the wedding. Ah, a woman's wedding to-do list: venue, dress, cake, photographer . . . and fertility doctor.

Always the planner, to assure that I would be able to have my fiancé's children; I decided I needed to go back to a reproductive specialist. I guess I should clarify that my first specialist had moved to Montana or Minnesota. Wherever it was, I never got a postcard.

I paid the new guy $535 for him to

explain basic sex-ed to me. Thank you very much. I got that one covered. He did at least tell me he saw no reason why I would not be pregnant within six months of being married. In fact, he even wanted me to go back on birth control for a few months to "jump start things." (I had not been on any birth control for a little over a year in order to start working on ovulating again.) At least being back on the pill helped me lose twelve pounds in three weeks which helped me fit into my wedding dress.

During the planning of the ceremony, I made sure the minister did not mention any presumptuous comments about my husband and I having children. That is always a pet peeve of mine at weddings, along with buffet style dinners.

The minute the honeymoon was over (Hello! I'm not going to conceive my child and then celebrate with a rum punch!), I went off birth control again, and we started "trying."

Trying
Chapter 2

"Trying." The alarming thing about that term is when someone tells you they are "trying," you inevitably get a mental picture of them and their partner having sex. No? Well, I do. What can I say? I must have a vivid and intrusive imagination.

Anyway, "trying" is not this exciting time of revisiting the sex life you had when the relationship was new. "Trying" starts out with working hard to have sex on the right days. Then it goes to making sure the two of you are having sex in precisely the right positions. Have you ever seen a woman go into a headstand immediately after sex? My husband has. Ever seen a woman prop her hips up with pillows for exactly twenty minutes after sex? My husband has. Unfortunately, my husband has seen a lot more creative and innovative methods of conceiving as well.

"Trying" means having to have sex, even after a hellacious fight. "Trying" means your husband knows way too much about your "egg whites." Trying is trying on a relationship.

* * *

Two weeks after the honeymoon, one week off birth control, we had dinner with my father-in-law:

I asked, "Guess what?"

He shouted, "You're pregnant!"

"Um, no, we went snorkeling," I replied.

That would be the first of hundreds of those awkward moments where I certainly was not going to say, "but we're trying."

But we were trying. We got married in January. (Refrain from any negative judgment on a winter wedding, because it was gorgeous. Snow wasn't an issue, and it was less expensive.) February, I had a sinus infection, so surely that was why I didn't get pregnant that month. Irrational, I know. March, hello period, but at least I was regular enough to have a period. April, I was going to turn 27 and not be pregnant. I still had plenty of time before the six months the specialist had given me were up.

May, this was all starting to get pretty frustrating. Side note: Mother's day is always so obnoxious for a woman trying to have a baby. Having been a social worker, what about all the children I've cared for whose mother's didn't care?

June, one more month and we had hit our deadline. July. Six months of trying. Not pregnant. Let's give it one more month. I was sure I would get pregnant one month past when the doctor said, just to teach me a little bit of faith and patience. Well, maybe two months past.

When I started my period in August, we decided it was time to call the doctor. I scheduled the appointment, and my husband scheduled off work. Three weeks later, and the appointment was the next day. I realized I had had not received the typical 24-hour notice call, and decided to call just to confirm. They had no record of my appointment. Three weeks of anticipation and nerves, just to be suspended.

The doctor did at least call, and we had a brief phone conversation discussing what to expect in initial testing. It sounded a little excessive, very invasive, and even more expensive. Pay to have my va-jay-jay power washed? Eek!

I also wasn't big on the doctor's vibe. If someone is going to be elbow deep inside of me, I'd like to think I could at least have a brief conversation about the weather . . . or vaginas . . . without being extremely annoyed.

Being the shop-a-holic that I am, I decided it was time to shop around for a new specialist. I found a place that someone I knew had success with, and it was significantly cheaper. I made an appointment. My husband and I finally had an appointment with a doctor to discuss infertility, 2 ½ months shy of our first anniversary.

Let's take that one in for a minute: Any woman who has sat in a fertility office understands that while there is the positive side of hoping you are one step closer to the child you are wanting, the reality is that it just really, really sucks.

I remember seven months before our wedding; I was late on my period. Being an obsessive early pregnancy tester, I took a pregnancy test. The results were a false positive.

I remember sobbing about how we had already paid all the deposits, but that it would be so tacky to be eight months pregnant in a wedding gown. Sob, sob, sob. What I would later have given for that pregnancy test to have been a true positive.

Most "responsible" women spend a decade or more of their lives on birth control, being so cautious to not be scorned by society for getting pregnant at an "unacceptable time." Now, that I wasn't pregnant at an "acceptable time," I felt more scorned than I could have ever imagined, for having to drag my husband to the doctors to confirm that I really was "damaged goods."

Missed Conception

On Your Marks, Get Set...
Chapter 3

I had made sure for our first fertility appointment together, that my husband and I looked "worthy" of being parents. I don't know what really constitutes as looking "worthy" of parenthood, but somehow my husband wearing a collared shirt and me doing my hair and make-up made me think the specialist would be a little more apt to help us.

The doctor was great, despite him telling me that I would need to go on Metformin again and that my hairy face wouldn't be fixed until I was done trying to have children. He also said not to already be considering in vitro fertilization (IVF), but to just think about Clomid and perhaps an intrauterine insemination (IUI).

One of the first specialists I initially saw told me Clomid would be all that was necessary, and while I knew my biological clock had ticked some in the past several years, I was confident that remained the case.

Now that my husband was in on the fertility regime with me, he became my "DH." Fertility chat boards love to use initials for EVERYTHING. DH is "dear husband." I will refer to him as DH from here on out, but feel free to substitute "dear husband" for "damned husband" if there are times where you know my hormones would have been thinking that instead.

* * *

I had quit my job to start an organizing business and had been a housewife for three weeks at the time of our appointment. I had walked 3 ½ miles every day during that time, limited my calories to 1200 a day and had still somehow managed to gain two pounds. Before this two pound weight gain, I had gained 30 pounds since our wedding. This was in addition to the 15 pounds I had gained from going off birth control the year before the wedding to try to start my body ovulating again. Do the math - it's scary! I was now at 198. I'm sure I tipped 200, but I refused to get back on the scale.

Then the Metformin began. Ever had the flu every day of your life? Well, that is what it is like for me, the 5ish percent or so who have nausea, diarrhea and bloating as side effects. As unpleasant as the Metformin was, I was desperately hoping it would help me lose some of the weight.

By the end of January, I had been on the Metformin for almost three months. I was still sick, no weight loss and oh yeah, no baby either. On top of that, the nausea from the Metformin, combined with already out-of-whack hormones, makes it really easy to convince yourself every month that you are pregnant and experiencing morning sickness.

All of January I was certain I was pregnant. My bank statements were riddled with purchases at the local grocery store for $6.99; the sale price of the generic pregnancy test.

I understand that I could have just waited for the dreaded period to eventually come, but who really does that? I also am aware of the argument for only buying the most expensive pregnancy tests. There is something less abrasive about not seeing the envied "+" verses the expensive brand's, "NOT

PREGNANT" written across the test. Ugh! Not to mention at the rate I was buying pregnancy tests, who could afford anything but the cheapies?

I went in for a blood test in the middle of January to see about some kind of levels that would indicate if I had ovulated. I had thought all of January that I was pregnant, but I came to find out that I hadn't even ovulated that month.

The next news from the fertility office was the doctor calling to let me know the results of more testing. Upon further review, numbers looked worse than originally thought. So the doctor recommended beginning Clomid and making sure to accompany it with an IUI. This fertility stuff was going to be more intense than anyone had expected.

Less than a half an hour later, I received another phone call. This time it was from my mother. My dad's lung cancer was back and had spread to his lymph nodes. The cancer would be aggressively terminal this time. His prognosis was about 8 months.

A lump formed in my throat to hold back the tears. Even if I got pregnant that second (which the fertility doctor had already made pretty clear would not be happening), I still would not get to see my dad interact with my child the way he had with my niece and nephew. I would not even get a picture of my dad holding my baby. My child wouldn't know my dad and would have lost a grandpa before he or she was even born.

Sadness overwhelmed me that day. It settled in to my bones and would affect me more and stay with me much longer than I would ever realize. It was a sadness that could only be half explained to others due to the decision to keep our infertility a secret.

Missed Conception

Alternative Method Month
Chapter 4

With the uphill battle getting steeper by hearing that we were definitely looking at needing the help of an IUI, I desperately searched for additional ways to boost our chances of fertility. We were now not only in a race against my biological clock, but against my dad's lack of time as well.

To ensure DH had Superman sperm, and I was doing all I could, we turned to holistic methods.

So the take-your-vitamins-like-they're-crack-cocaine campaign began for DH. He religiously took COQ10, Fish Oil, Dandelion Root and multivitamins every day. I continued with my prenatal vitamins and other occasional supplements.

Other than a stint in Key West, we

significantly decreased all alcohol intake as well. I had read a study that showed even two alcoholic drinks a day could decrease a woman's fertility by as much as 60%. Saying that I was giving up alcohol because of Lent, helped to avoid the nagging, "Why aren't you drinking? Are you pregnant?"

Still not wanting to think I would need Clomid, I decided to do the alternative method of acupuncture. I am deathly afraid of needles. Actually, as I am assuming any woman who has gone through fertility does, I have now grown accustom to needles. So I should say, I *was* deathly afraid of needles. Having 30+ needles poked all over your body, even in your ears, is not what I would consider pleasant, but I do believe there were benefits.

One benefit of acupuncture was it jump-started my weight loss. I had three sessions within about five weeks, and I lost 22 pounds. For the first time in seven years I was able to lose weight!

I also started to try doing better with Yoga. Perhaps if I could "open my pelvic region," I'd be preggers. I was on a positive path.

Vitamins, acupuncture, yoga, a

massage, no alcohol, and four fertility books later, I was ready to finally expedite the process and bite the bullet . . . or anyone's head off, while now on Clomid.

Missed Conception

Round 1, Round 2
Chapter 5

By March, I had decided to start Clomid. There were plenty of horror stories to be heard about Clomid: weight gain, raging hormones, vomiting, etc. My first time taking it, I only noticed that my vision was blurred one night; I was a little light-headed and incredibly tired. Others would probably say I was a little volatile too, but I'm not asking them.

One "slight" indication that perhaps my hormones were causing me to be a little out of character (even though at times I do have a heightened baseline of the crazies), was on a day when I decided to watch *The Ellen DeGeneres Show*. Ellen's guests on the show were a family who had adopted four boys from Africa.

About twenty minutes later, DH walked through the front door from work and found me sobbing hysterically. I was online looking into the best rate for plane tickets to Africa so I could visit the orphanage.

Even through the tears, there was an acknowledgement that my emotions might be a little over the top. That's the thing about hormones; you can be laughing and sobbing in the same few seconds . . . and needing to book a ticket to Africa!

A week or so after taking the Clomid, I went to the doctor's. The doctor reported that my follicles had not grown and told me to come back in a few days to see if there was any change.

Two days later, there was still no growth. In addition, I had been feeling severe pain in the middle-right of my back. And, oh the burps. I could burp louder and longer than any burly man out there. The doctor said it sounded like I had gastritis and wanted to be cautious to avoid peptic ulcers. This meant that we would now have to balance the length of my fertility attempts with what my intestines, liver and gallbladder could sustain under the medication. Fantastic.

The intestinal problems were annoying; however, it was crushing to know that I had finally succumbed to fertility meds, and my body still was not positively responding. Although, when it comes to fertility struggles, what is crushing one month seems menial compared to the disappointments that can follow.

* * *

In the interval between Clomid treatments, I went in to be fitted for a bridesmaid's dress. I have to be the only woman (besides every other woman going through this roller coaster), to leave David's Bridal with a dress that was too loose in the stomach. I surely was going to be pregnant in two months and if not showing already, feeling bloated and needing the extra room.

* * *

Round 2: Clomid. This time there was uncontrollable crying even strung throughout normal conversation:

Me: (to DH): "Would you like more, (sob, sob, sob), salad?"

DH: Uh, ok, what's wrong?

Me: "I don't know. This salad just makes me cry. I don't know why I'm crying, but I can't (sob, sob, sob) stop."

I also had *extreme* bloating. No exaggeration, I now knew what my body would look like if I were to ever be five months pregnant.

These more extreme side effects were probably due to my dose having been doubled which was a level the specialist didn't seem necessarily comfortable with. He suggested we try this dosage once before looking in to other medications due to my gastritis and the increased risk of twins. Because I have the need to overly process with people, I explained to the doctor that I was okay with conceiving twins. I had experience, and I knew what I would be getting myself into.

The hesitation I once had over having twins had disappeared. I used to worry life with twins would always be in "go" mode (because I hate the term survival mode when dealing with babies), and that it would be hard to cherish every second of their infancy. Now, the chance of twins seemed to be the best opportunity to be able to be closer to the size of family I always wanted without fertility treatments always looming over my head. Fertility thoughts may not always be proper, but they are honest.

I went into the doctor's office; certain with the double dose, there would be good news. Nope. The follicles were all still too small. Come back in two days. Pay for two visits. The news was identical to the month before.

What if I was starting the Clomid on the wrong day? My period wasn't exactly the most by-the-book event. Worse yet, what if the Clomid just wasn't going to work? I decided to start a journal to my baby. I wanted them to know how I longed for him or her.

4/24/12

Dear Baby,

It's getting so hard to be patient waiting for you. I had another disappointing doctor's visit yesterday. My body just isn't responding to the medicine. I know you will come someday, but my anxieties sometimes let the fear of never being a mother overwhelm me. Your daddy says God just needs more time to make such an extra special baby.

I'm almost finished painting the spare bedroom, and it is fun for me to think about how I would decorate it as a nursery. I've already started looking at nursery decorations and furniture. I have daddy talk with me about baby names too.

If you're a girl, Elizabeth Faye will probably be your name. I will call you Eliza. It's important to me that a girl has a name that will suit her in the professional world. Eliza sounds southern to me, and Faye is after your maternal grandfather's family.

Boy names have been a lot more challenging. Daddy wants a Jr. It's important to me that you set your own legacy (not to mention it would be confusing having two of the same name in one home). I also worry that if we were ever blessed with two boys, the second might feel left out. I love the name Graham, but Daddy isn't a fan. Vincent (Vince), Jack and Abram are the others we like. Oh, and William.

My dad, of course your

grandpa, probably won't live to see you. He will be your guardian angel though and has supported Daddy and me in our decision to do fertility. He cuts newspaper articles out about medical advancements, etc. in the hopes you will come to us soon. The stuffed bunny I bought to keep him company during hospital visits will be in your nursery at his request.

I just can't imagine how amazing it will feel to watch my belly grow with you in it and then feel you in my arms.

Love,
Mommy

Two days following the last doctor visit, my husband and I went in for another appointment. DH had already taken the day off thinking that would have been when the IUI was scheduled. The doctor excitedly announced that I had one follicle that was 17mm. It was go time!

4/25/12

Dear Baby,

33

I had your dad come with me today to my doctor's appointment, worried we would receive more bad news and need to decide alternative paths to conceiving you. The doctor's face lit up as he was doing my ultrasound, and it turns out my body has decided to try to make it time to plan for your arrival! We will go through the procedure on Saturday.

After the doctor's, we immediately went to Home Depot to get the rest of my painting supplies. I want to have my projects finished before Saturday, because I worry about painting while pregnant.

I'm trying my best to do everything right to give you the best chance at optimum health. I didn't even have my Diet Coke today - BIG sacrifice! I also scheduled more acupuncture appointments to increase our chances of this procedure being a success.

I've already cried tears of joy, just at the hope today has given me.

Daddy is so happy too. I must remember God's planning and timing is better than mine.

Love,
Mommy

Missed Conception

IUI Oh My
Chapter 6

4/27/12

Dear Baby,

Tomorrow is our IUI. I am _so_ nervous! Yesterday, I gave myself a shot in the belly (actually, I did it twice just to make sure I got out all the medicine), and today I did my acupuncture. Now, I am saying my prayers and keeping my fingers crossed!

I saw a baby tonight that was only a month old and had brown hair. It made me think of what you might look like. I can't wait to have you here, to hold you, read to you and just be with you.

I know there is only a 13-15%

chance tomorrow will work, but I feel your arrival is near. I desperately want that to be so. Sometimes, (ok, a lot of the time), I find myself wondering why we are having to go through this challenge when there are bad people who can have children easily. A question to ask God! I know it will all be worth it in the end. In the mean time, it has brought Daddy and I closer, and we will be that much more excited for your arrival!

Love,
Mommy

The night before the IUI, my nerves skyrocketed. The next day, potentially, would be the first day that I was a mom. The alarm clock could not sound soon enough.

The alarm didn't have to sound. I was dressed and ready to go far before it went off. We were on our way.

DH and I sat in a separate room at the doctor's office, waiting for him to give his "sample." Let's just pause on this one to rant a moment: Women, we are amazing. *Amazing!* We get poked and prodded, gain weight, lose weight, lose all control over our emotions, vomit, have hot flashes, nausea, dizziness, and so much more just to get pregnant . . . and the boys get a bottle of lotion and their option of dirty magazines.

Anyway, watching men come out of the "exam" rooms is a little unsettling. Watching one of the men come out and look at the palm of his hand was downright disturbing.

Then a new worry came slamming into my anxiety ridden mind. WHAT IF THEY MIXED UP THE "SAMPLES?" I definitely needed to oversee this situation like a buzzard on road kill.

The crotchety old lady behind the desk turned out to be a real problem in allowing me to hang out and supervise the situation. So, after DH's "task" was finished, we went out for breakfast. As we were being seated, I realized our table would be right next to a baby. Ugh! They are everywhere! Enjoying a nice meal out is the time to do exactly that, enjoy – not be highly annoyed by the kids next to you or even worse, stare longingly at something you want but don't yet have.

Lucky for me, this baby was one of the ugliest babies out there. DH thinks I'm awful for thinking some babies are ugly, but ugly people start as ugly babies, so it is what it is.

We finished up our breakfast and headed back to the doctor's office to pick up the "sample." The crotchety old woman was still planted at the front desk. Obviously, she forgot that she was dealing with a woman pumped full of hormones.

After standing in front of Ms. Crotchety for several minutes with no acknowledgement, I went ahead and inquired about our sample. She proceeded to tell me that it was not ready and asked for my appointment time. I explained our appointment was at 10 a.m., to which she replied that we were early.

Do *not* cross me and my time. If I do one thing well, it is time management. "IT IS 9:52. WE WERE TOLD TO PICK UP THE SAMPLE TEN MINUTES BEFORE OUR 10:00 APPOINTMENT. I BEGAN STANDING AT YOUR DESK AT 9:48, AT WHICH TIME I WAS TWO MINUTES EARLY, BUT I AM NOW TWO MINUTES LATE FOR MY APPOINTMENT!"

Didn't this woman know the early bird gets the sperm?! It was time for me to take a water fountain break so I could reign myself in.

Now I had really done it. So much for ensuring I didn't get one of those goofball's "samples." If servers spit in people's food, what could this woman have done to the genetics of my future child?

DH walked out shortly after with his "sample" in a brown paper bag like a proud first grader with his first bagged lunch. Oh my.

After time conflicts were resolved with my doctor's office (I knew that woman was going to throw us off schedule!), we were called back. I was up on the exam table and so nervous, I thought I was either going to pass out or scream. Oh, nope, just more tears.

In came the doctor, and out came the incredibly long straw thing. I was told it was going to be like a Pap test . . . .

First my vajayjay was cranked open with a vice grip thing. No exaggeration when I say "cranked," as I'm pretty sure the doctor literally was cranking something open to dilate me enough to have this child nine months from now.

Next, the doctor looked at the numbers on the paper attached to the brown paper bag. He said the numbers all looked good – thank you vitamin campaign!

The doctor then sucked up the sample, inserted the straw thing, and HOLY SHIT! What the hell was that? I jumped, as it felt a hornet had been released inside me. Then it was over. My legs were propped up high, and my hopes were up even higher.

When Life Hands You Lemons
Chapter 7

4/30/12

Dear Baby,

Saturday I was a nervous wreck! I think I slept about 4 hours the night before. Daddy's numbers were healthy, and my procedure went pretty smoothly. So now, we just wait - and wait - and wait.

I had a bachelorette party Saturday night and a Red's game with friends on Sunday. Not having a glass of wine raised people's suspicions, but we have only told a very few about our plans for you.

Your uncle is super excited and hopeful for us.

It's been a week without Diet Coke, and I've cut down on my caffeine. I passed up the sushi the other night too. I'm feeling tired and crampy. I've also began craving pasta, powdered sugar doughnuts and LEMON ANYTHING. This could easily just be my crazy hormones or all the medicine, but I'm hopeful it's signs of the first three days of your being.

Love,
Mommy

After the IUI, I went home and relaxed for a couple of hours. Then I was off to be the designated driver for a bachelorette party.

The night started with a wine tasting. The other girls said they felt badly for drinking in front of me, but I truly didn't care. I was so content to know that the beginning of my baby could be forming.

The next day I was at a baseball game, and snuck O'Douls in a regular beer cup to avoid the questions . . . only three people asked instead of thirteen.

I had experienced a little cramping on Saturday and Sunday. By Monday it felt like a bowling ball was in my stomach, a very heavy pulling. I took it easy for a couple of days, and all cramping went away. What came, were the cravings.

Lemons, lemon cake, lemons, lemon cookies, lemons, lemonade, lemon sorbet, lemons, lemon water. Did I mention I usually don't even like a small slice of lemon in my tea? Just seeing something yellow made my mouth water for lemons.

The mind is such a powerful thing. Once the cravings kicked in, not once did I consciously think about how the hamster hormones I had injected in my stomach would cause me to emulate pregnancy. I was convinced I was pregnant.

When DH and I went to a hoity-toity café, and I was too sick to eat my Italian food (unheard of for me), I was even more sure that I was pregnant. After lunch, we were walking around the outside eating area, and I had to lean against a tree as I dry heaved in front of everyone eating. I was elated. This had to be my first bout with true morning sickness. I felt like I was on top of the world - while under the tree puking.

* * *

05/3/12

Dear Baby,

 Today is the first day since the IUI that I haven't felt any cramping. I'm worried that it didn't work, since I'm no longer feeling anything. I've looked on the internet to try to find some answers, but I think I'm just going to have to learn patience. I've been trying not to get my hopes up, but that simply isn't possible.

 "Our light and momentary troubles are achieving for us an eternal glory that far outweighs them all." (2 Corinthians 4:17).

 If I just knew that this was all momentary, and that I will experience being a mother, it would be a lot easier to deal with. I'm becoming so resentful that we aren't able to have a child naturally.

 I desperately hope you are growing in my belly right now.

Love,
Mommy

One week down at this point, in the two week wait. The infamous "two-week wait" is arguably one of the longest periods of someone's life. Fourteen days, in my case 16 due to office scheduling, to find out if the IUI worked. It was made clear not to take a home pregnancy test, due to the injection being in your system and causing a false positive. So it truly was going to be two weeks.

To get me through the second week, I began planning the nursery. Premature planning, I think not. I was convinced I was pregnant, and this was something I wanted to do a long time ago. For a boy, it would be a sailor theme: navy accents, whale rug, personalized anchor wall décor. For a girl, I would have a neutral and soft pink cherry blossom theme.

So the first week of waiting started off with general themes for the nursery. By the end of the second week, I had diaper bags, mobiles, cribs, gliders, sheet sets, and everything else picked out. Basically, I had registered, sans registry.

That Friday, I sat scrapbooking on the

living room floor, again watching *The Ellen DeGeneres Show.* I found myself to be so content. That particular episode was in honor of expecting mothers to celebrate the upcoming Mother's Day that was two days away. I took mental notes on certain products and watched with my hand on my stomach (not much scrapbooking was done), thinking about how I soon would have a pregnant belly like everyone one in the audience.

After the show was over, I got back to scrapbooking. I needed to get all pictures organized by the time my life was consumed with the baby and thousands of more pictures!

Then I felt again what seemed like premenstrual cramps. This cramping had happened once the day before and once even the day before that. Although every time I had felt this, I was lifting something heavy. It had to be implementation cramping, but my involuntary reaction to pray and pray hard told me I knew there could be another, less desirable explanation.

T.K.O.
Chapter 8

Friday evening, technically the last day of my two week wait, I went to the bathroom and realized I had spotted. I had read about this on the internet. By the way, I'm a doctor, just ask WebMD. It had to be implementation bleeding; not my period.

By the time I walked back to the living room, I collapsed in tears. Why couldn't this have happened on Monday before my appointment? Why couldn't I have had just one Mother's Day with the hope that I was pregnant?

When DH got home that night, it was even more devastating. DH is optimistic almost to a fault. He is always the light at the end of the tunnel. He never allows time for negative thoughts and always believes that winning the lottery, a sunny day, and pregnancy are right around the corner. That night, I think the reality came crashing in on him.

I will never forget when he said, "The thing is, I would have considered us lucky. To watch you give yourself shots, quit your job, be sick every day, pay all this money, and try for almost two years. If we had gotten pregnant with the first IUI, I would have considered us lucky. Here some people just have sex. Things like that just don't happen for us." Surprised by this side of him I had never seen before, I somehow was able to be the strong one that night.

The next day, I was still just spotting. Hope conquers reality, and I was back on the internet, madly searching for a website that would tell me I still had reason to believe that I was pregnant. Between the internet's many message boards and me, the consensus was that the HCG shot only stays in your system a maximum of 10 days. I was off to buy a pregnancy test.

I know that I am great at convincing myself at things I want to believe, but I do not hallucinate. There was a blue line in the pregnancy window. Snap. Picture taken. I was on my way to show DH. I was helping out that night at the restaurant where he works, so I pulled him out of the kitchen and showed him the picture.

DH admitted the line was there but said he wasn't going to get his hopes up. That was okay, because my hopes were high enough for the both of us.

The next morning: Mother's Day. I had awoken to the realization my pad was soaked. It had not been implementation bleeding. It was a period. It was not a positive pregnancy test. It was a cruel joke.

DH and I have a tradition of celebrating Mother's Day and Father's Day for each other anyway. We celebrate it for the job we do as an Aunt and Uncle, and we celebrate it for what we have already done for our future child. We celebrate it, because it is a hard day, and we need support.

We celebrated that Mother's Day with going out for a glazed doughnut, and then me needing to go home to cry - blubbering tears the entire way to the doughnut shop wasn't enough. Later, we went out to dinner. Instead of more crying, I decided to go to the bar, drink excessively and tell every woman I saw "Happy Vajayjay Day."

I didn't want to take anything away

from all the amazing mothers out there who are working diligently to raise the human beings that will someday have a positive impact on humanity. However, this particular Mother's Day, I also didn't want to take anything away from my pity party.

* * *

Reveling in one's depression is a luxury that I do suggest from time to time indulging in, but only for a short, very short period of time. Perhaps an afternoon would do.

I decided I should get almost a month to indulge in depression. In my defense, and every other woman out there undergoing fertility treatments, hormones are a powerful thing.

The week after we realized we weren't pregnant, was the week that it seemed like the rest of the world realized that they *were* pregnant. Two days after Mother's Day, two different people came up to DH and me, and announced they were pregnant. The day after that, I saw a woman whom I hadn't seen since her wedding almost a year after mine. She was already at least five months pregnant. Ugh! I quickly headed the other direction in the grocery store to avoid having to say "Congratulations."

That week was also one of the hardest on our relationship. I am a big believer that even in devastation, positive things can arise. DH and I became a lot closer during this fertility phase. I have learned to trust him more with my weaknesses, and he has become supportive in ways I never thought possible. With that being said, everyone has their breaking point.

God made the world in only seven days, and it *only* took me seven days to figure out how to articulate what I was feeling. It was a week's worth of drinking and a lot of screaming. I wanted to scream loud enough that everyone would know my pain.

Eventually I had slammed enough doors to finally break down and beg my husband. I begged him over and over to just tell me how mad he was at me for not being pregnant. He wouldn't do it.

That was the day that I wore the bridesmaid's dress with the now unneeded room in the stomach. That was the day we decided to take a break from it all.

Missed Conception

A Break After the Breaking Point
Chapter 9

5/22/12

Dear Baby,

I have been too sad to write. On Mother's Day I realized the IUI hadn't worked. Daddy was more upset than I have ever seen him. My oldest friend told me tonight, "I know someday you will be a mother. Nobody is more maternal than you. This is something you've desired your whole life. When we were growing up, no other kid even had more baby dolls than you."

I just feel lost when I'm not

raising a child, but I also am at a point where I don't want to be around kids unless they are finally my own.

We have decided to take a month or two off from the fertility treatments. . . . The other meds are too much. I need a break. . . .

Having faith in God, means also having faith in His timing.

Love,
Mommy

Taking a break may mean easing up on the medicines and doctor visits, but it does not necessarily mean taking your mind off of fertility. There is not a day that goes by that I don't think about wanting a baby. Even when I get to do positive things I wouldn't be able to do as a mother, like sleeping in late, I think about what it would be like to have woken up to a baby.

One significant difference during our "break time" was our sex life. Of course, I still had an app on my Iphone to chart my ovulation . . . or when a person with a text-book ovary would ovulate. Of course, I still hoped every time that we had sex I would miraculously conceive; however for me, the pressure was temporarily off.

I don't know if it was the hormones trying to figure themselves out or the risqué, romance novel I was reading. Either way, we actually had a sex life again and not just a trying-to-conceive life. DH noticed it too. . . . Oh boy, did he notice!

Also during the break, I found myself feeling more pressure to start sharing with people what we had been going through. It was like I was coming up for air, and needed to gather support in case I started feeling like I was drowning when the treatments started again.

DH repeatedly said, "I just don't like to talk about it. I don't think it's anyone else's business. It's your body though, do what you want."

In an ideal world, I would have agreed. Actually, in an ideal world, I would agree with DH about more things in general. In reality though, some people I felt deserved to know.

One person I really wanted to share our journey with was my father-in-law. As mentioned earlier, he was the first to ask when we were going to have a baby. Unlike some of the nosey people I knew, I know he was asking out of anticipation and excitement.

Telling him was not as simple as just wanting to though. I knew that once I told him, it was likely everyone in DH's family would hear about it. I also felt that the news needed to come from DH. More importantly, I felt my father-in-law was already disappointed that we had not given him grandchildren. Did I really want to burden him with the disappointment that it was not an easy possibility?

Because of so much confusion and confliction on how to communicate our experience, I decided to start a support group. I felt this would be my answer to unwind the frustrations by being able to talk to other women who were in the exact situation as me. So I went on Craigslist and posted the offer that if anyone with PCOS or fertility problems wanted to chat, email me and perhaps we could all meet at a coffee shop.

I received four replies. Four replies out of an entire tri-state area. That was ok, I was still excited. Four women plus me definitely equaled a group.

The women who had replied all shared a little about themselves. One didn't have a car, and one lived outside of the city. So I decided we could start with a support group over e-mail.

I very briefly shared my story and my excitement to be able to hear from other women about suggestions, struggles and successes. I never heard a response from any of the four again. Ouch.

The support group obviously was not a hit. Journaling to my future child definitely had been helping and kept me focused on the goal and trying to be positive. It was the interaction with other women who I knew were out there, that I really wanted to have and needed. If they didn't come to me, I would come to them via this book.

So I began to type. I might as well dialogue all my thoughts and mood swings with my laptop. As I did, I began to feel a calling and a purpose - both of which I hadn't felt in years. It made me wonder how many more chapters of infertility I would have.

When supportive husbands were not enough and Craigslist support groups didn't respond, maybe a woman could take my book off the shelf and find solace in knowing someone else was out there crying, hoping, booking tickets to African orphanages, craving lemons, longing and learning. Infertility does not have to be so isolating.

* * *

Fortunately, there were ways infertility was being more exposed every day. There were currently three shows on TV that I knew of, and DVRd religiously, discussing couples' struggles with trying to have a baby. I picked up a magazine the other day and saw where another woman announced she was now "trying everything" to have a child.

I feel so blessed that I am meeting this obstacle in an age where medical technology is capable of assisting and voices are starting to speak out. The more voices there are, the more ears will hear that infertility is not a situation of needing to relax . One comment that is consistently made to me is, "Well, it will happen when you just relax. Just give up, and you'll get pregnant."

First of all, I will *never* give up. Secondly, if it were a matter of merely relaxing, I would have just scheduled an afternoon at the spa. (I've tried that too and didn't leave pregnant. Imagine that.)

This is a medical condition that has given me the prognosis of as little as a 1%-2%

chance of DH and me conceiving on our own. Infertility in a woman is a medical condition that needs awareness, support and fundraising just like any other medical condition.

Despite starting to see infertility discussed on TV and in magazines, it was not being discussed at family dinners or in casual conversation at social events. When someone on TV is driving to a fertility doctor in their Range Rovers with their checkbook in their Hermes bag and their Prada sunglasses covering their tears, a lot of the raw reality is hidden by reality TV.

If I could afford a Hermes bag, I probably would not have spent so much of my "break" worried about money. God has always given me just enough in my bank account, but that doesn't stop a worrier from worrying. It is one thing to know that you might not have enough money to take the vacation you've been hoping for, but when you start seeing every purchase as taking away from your chance to have a child, things get stressful.

Missed Conception

Kayak or Kids

Chapter 10

DH lost his wedding ring . . . in the mouth of a large mouth bass to be exact. At least it was insured. He is now wearing the cheapest ring we could find, and the rest of the insurance check went to the have-a-baby fund.

The fishing incident was actually great timing. It had been seven months after quitting my job, and I was still sick every morning – with fertility meds, not a baby. We had already used ¾ of the money we received from our wedding on treatments.

This is when one going through infertility begins to see every past purchase, from wedding to vacation to groceries, as having no purpose but to have depleted the baby fund. I needed to get another job, sick or not.

In the meantime, I had a close acquaintance go on and on about how the one thing she knew for certain in her life was that she made "the most beautiful babies." She proceeded to tell me that if DH and I ever were to find ourselves having trouble conceiving, she would sell us one of her eggs. Despite all the financial worries I was having, how to buy an egg from this woman never would cross my mind.

However, there were plenty of other financial burdens crossing my mind. Writing out the check to pay for the last $500 on the IUI caused so much inner confliction. I would pay anything to have a child. Unfortunately, our income wasn't a "pay anything" income.

I hated giving money to the doctor for a procedure that didn't even work. I hated that other people used their money to start college funds for their children, to buy a nicer house, or to take a family vacation. We were spending all of our savings just in an attempt to conceive.

It seemed other people only spent money on a nice dinner and a bottle of wine to conceive . . . and still others seemed to be the type that bought a Forty and a bag of pot before they conceived. I had to stop comparing myself to the "others." Theodore Roosevelt was so wise to say, "Comparison is the thief of joy."

Anyway, DH (damned husband in this conversation) came home the night after I paid our fertility bill and announced that he had been saving for a kayak. I didn't respond gently.

A kayak! Here I am selling my clothes to the consignment store for a little cash, and DH wants to buy a kayak? Alright, I was selling my clothes, because I hadn't been a size 8 in quite some time. Still, he had the audacity to want to spend our "baby money" on a kayak?

DH was as supportive as a husband could be with the fertility process. However, in moments like this, it was clear a man just doesn't hear the ticking of a biological clock as loudly as a woman.

* * *

When one aspect of my life seems out of control (i.e. finances and fertility), I feel an incredible need to take control in another area. I was sure there were inexpensive things I could do to get pregnant. I just hadn't tried hard enough. Back to exploring holistic thoughts and alternative approaches.

First off, I had been without my Diet Coke for two months. The entire "aspartame is liquid birth control" was something I had studied. The fact that I was a Coke addict, in the Diet Coke sense, was my new reason why I wasn't pregnant yet. I actually swore off all aspartame which happens to be in a lot more than I had realized.

It is kind of ironic swearing off aspartame, excessive wine, not even taking Advil during an IUI, and being so cautious in general about what was entering my system when here I was on fertility drugs. I had injected hamster hormones in my body (the HCG shot) and God knows what other unnatural chemicals, but now I was going to blame Diet Coke for my problems?

Every once in awhile, I remembered to cut myself some slack. If crack addicts could get pregnant, I could have a sip of Diet Coke.

For the days I did cut myself slack, I had my vitamins as back-up. Since I was off of Clomid, I was taking an herb called Vitex. It's from the Chaste Tree. Why is a drug that is supposed to enhance ovulation regularity and make a woman more fertile named after abstinence? There was research on those trusty message boards and the vitex label said it had been used by women for thousands of years. That was enough evidence to convince me.

I also began taking Dandelion Root to help my liver detoxify and handle the Metformin. I continued taking my prenatal vitamins and added fish oil and CoQ10 to the mixture as well. I am not sure if all of these herbs should be taken together, but during the "break," it was my turn to put my WEBMD doctorate to the test.

Thirdly, I continued to try to do non-processed foods and stick to mostly organic. Organic milk was a must. Fertility books had advised that I try to do a serving of whole milk a day. The acupuncturist suggested berries were the trick due to the antioxidants. My blender was busy pureeing up berry smoothies with whole yogurt.

Fourth form of control: I must not be getting pregnant, because I am too fat. Even though the Metformin had helped me lose 10% of my body weight, that isn't that much when you start out in the 200 ballpark. I was now at 180 and really wanting to lose another 20 pounds to feel like I had control of my weight. For the first time since a brief stint in high school, I made exercise a part of my daily routine. Sure there were days I skipped, but for the most part I had made the treadmill and yoga a positive habit that I hope I will continue throughout the rest of my life. See, positive things do come from fertility struggles.

At the end of the day, none of these attempts seemed to be making a difference in the baby department. So I did what any other sane woman would do. I ordered a sage stick to ward off the evil spirits in my home that were preventing the stork from getting to my uterus. Hey, desperate times, desperate measures.

Namaste . . . Or Not
Chapter 11

In a 105-degree room surrounded by perfect bodies in cute little work-out outfits, was me: drenched in sweat, muscles shaking, hoping I didn't pass out or puke while trying to do Bikram Yoga.

Hm, childbirth would probably be far worse than this. As an extremist, I went to the extreme when I said I was going to try harder at yoga. From a few breathing DVDs, I then signed up for this 90 minute class that couldn't end fast enough.

My coupon for the class was expiring in two weeks, and I sure was not going to pay $20 a class to endure this. Maybe I would switch to a less strenuous yoga.

Two more weeks was also when I was supposed to start my period. DH had been asking if I was ready to start treatments again. I had put him off with the thought that I probably would not be ready until August. I was finally feeling back to normal; now back to fertility?

Part of me was excited about trying aggressively again to have a baby. Another part of me was more scared than before.

Ignorance is bliss, and I was no longer ignorant. As soon as I began considering it, I thought about things I would have to rearrange for the remainder of the summer to accommodate fertility appointments, etc. I also realized that I was still struggling with giving up the hope that we would magically, naturally become pregnant.

We celebrated DH's 30th birthday, and the pressure of time seemed prominent. I did not want to put off fertility treatments, put off having a baby, if July could be the month that we conceived.

I had not lost the weight or saved the money I had wanted to before we started more treatments, but I had a nagging feeling telling me it was time to start again. My nagging feelings are hard to distinguish between my

OCD and what could be Divine Intervention.

* * *

At the end of the brutal yoga class, I was always euphoric to hear the instructor walk out of the classroom as she said, "Namaste." I realized this was a term used in yoga, but my only translation of it was, "Thank God I didn't die from exhaustion. Time to get in air conditioning and figure out what my caloric intake is going to be as a reward." One night I looked up the meaning to discover I should have perhaps been interpreting it more accurately as, "to bow to your core self."

This yoga saying might have a point. With all other extrinsic fertility factors aside, my "core self" would be the most important thing in going through more fertility treatments. In order to muster the endurance I needed for these treatments, I needed to not focus on my future baby, but to focus on who I was with or without that baby.

My identity did not solely exist within the attempts to have a baby. Even when I became a mother, my identity should not solely exist within motherhood. I needed to actively and consciously reclaim the things I enjoyed, resume my productivity in society and cease the negative self talk I had grown so accustomed to doing. By focusing on this, I would not be trying less to conceive, but instead trying more to remember who I was.

This was probably going to be easier said than done ….

* * *

As predicted, rediscovering my "core self" was already hitting a road block. I had made the decision to start again with fertility treatments. I called the doctor and was told I would be put on Femara instead of Clomid.

 Femara is a cancer drug for post-menopausal breast cancer patients. It was supposed to work when Clomid didn't. I wasn't sure what to think about the doctor having already given up on Clomid for me or the thought of taking a cancer drug without having cancer. I was excited though, to have hope in a different drug. My prescriptions were called into the pharmacy, and we were set to start treatments whenever my period started.

After I got off the phone, I went to the bathroom only to discover that for the first time ever, I was having an early period. Well, that would explain my bitchiness and overeating the past couple of days.

The problem was I no longer could start treatments this month, because it would have me starting in the middle of our only summer trip. I was not going to be on a new medication in someone else's home.

If I had just started three days later, everything would have been as planned. Now we would be resuming treatments in August not July.

Then it sunk in. This month was my last month to get pregnant in order to have a baby before I turned 29.

For anyone who has gone through fertility, you understand that your life goes into total calendar mode. If I started my period today, I need to start my new medication on Wednesday which means I should be ovulating by the 12th. Doctor visits will be on the 12th and maybe the 14th too since my ovaries like to get sassy. If everything goes well, then I should have my IUI on the 16th which means I need to get my Ovidrel shot on the 15th. Two weeks later, we will find out when I hopefully get to put my due date on the calendar.

Oh, and how exciting if it does work. That would mean I won't be nine months pregnant in the middle of summer, and that my baby won't have a winter birthday where they always have to do indoor parties.

The fixation on the calendar had quickly replaced the goal to focus more on my "core self." Every month going through that calendar in your head, and adjusting it to fit each cycle, can really take its toll after a while. I was obsessed. Perhaps instead of focusing on my "core self," I'd start with trying to discard my "calendar-self."

Struggling Blessings

Chapter 12

6/8/12

Dear Baby,

I read a quote the other day that said, "Before your greatest miracle, come your greatest obstacles."

God keeps telling me, "It will happen." But when? How many treatments? How many kids will I get to have? HOW MUCH WILL WE HAVE TO GO THROUGH?

Daddy and I were discussing what kind of parents we want to be the other night. My desire is that *when the day comes that I have my own child, I will be a mother that helps him or her reach their utmost potential no matter what that potential may be. . . .*

. . . Hopefully, baby blessings will come our way!

Love,
Mommy

The mere fact that DH and I had discussions on what kind of parents we wanted to be before we even conceived was one of the many blessings about infertility. Yes, as much as I gripe about infertility, there are blessings that can arise from it. Our lives as parents have been so planned which has also allowed for our parenting to be so anticipated, wanted and carefully considered.

Conversations over parenting and other aspects of fertility have done something amazing to morph DH and my relationship. Always the woman who wants to appear independent with a tough outer shell, I have found myself needing a shoulder to cry on and learning a healthy dependence on DH. He has become protective of me and opened himself up to conversations about emotions I never thought I would hear him discuss.

You can talk until you are blue in the face about being a parent, but having experience with children is invaluable. While I need no lessons on how to change a diaper, feedings, behavioral management, etc., I do need a lesson on patience. To be a good mom, you have to be patient. Having troubles conceiving has also taught me patience in ways I would otherwise never have learned. I suppose patience really is a virtue.

While we are talking about virtues, I'll spill the beans on an obvious vice of mine: judging others.

Sometimes, I am not the only one judging. I have had a lot of judgment placed on me by others for not working full time while doing fertility. I know people work and do fertility, but for the time being, I am blessed with the luxury of not having to do so. The people who have judged me have also been the people who do not know about our infertility struggles. This has brought such awareness to me of how I judge others when I usually have no clue of what their situation may be.

I am by no means saying I have conquered the habit of judging others. I will probably always struggle to not judge.

Not judging others still remains a challenge in my personal life as well. When my father's cancer reoccurred, I kept my opinion to myself. My opinion though, was that he should not do chemotherapy and radiation. If it was imminent that it was his time to go, why should he spend what little time he did have taking on more suffering? How could I feel this way about my dad's decision when I would never stand for people questioning my decision to do fertility treatments?

Even though I am not tolerant of others questioning my fertility treatments, it still happens. When people really want to put some oomph behind their interrogations, they bring up the religious side.

There is the inevitable debate out there about the ethics behind fertility treatments. "If it were God's will, wouldn't I already be pregnant?" While questions are crucial, that particular question is a dangerous one. It can lead to placing a lot of blame on God. I would rather believe that if God made Mary the Mother of Jesus through Immaculate Conception, what fertility miracle does He have in store for me?

I have done a lot of reflection and had many conversations throughout the years about where I would draw the line with fertility in order to coincide with my spiritual beliefs. What was I doing to my body? Is any of this going to affect my child in ways science has yet to know? Is there a larger explanation for why we are going through this? What happened to the girl who sat in the college bioethics class who thought that people should adopt instead of considering fertility?

That girl was yours truly, and the reality is that girl learned. I knew adoption is an incredible, amazing experience that is beyond enriching. I learned it is also expensive, lengthy and complicated. I also learned that perhaps the world is not as black and white as the pages in a book – especially if you are the main character in the book.

My desire for a child knows no limits or boundaries. With that being said, fertility treatments do not oppose my spiritual beliefs. In fact, I think quite the opposite. Spirituality is an organic thing that grows as one grows in life experiences.

Going through infertility has helped me grow in my spirituality by seeking answers, comfort, and hope. Psalms 37:4 says, "Delight yourself in the Lord, and he will give you the desires of your heart." I don't know what the future holds, but I know that in the future, I will hold my baby.

Part Two

Missed Conception

Here We Go Again
Chapter 13

I was headed out to a pool party when I started my period a week early. Instead of stopping at the store for the daiquiri mix I was looking forward to, I picked up my Femara. As much as you try to plan around fertility, you just can't.

Femara is not begun until the third day of your period, but I liked to have my medicine on hand. You never know when your entire neighborhood might start doing fertility and need the exact same medicine, leaving all the pharmacies with a Femara shortage.

By the next day, I realized that I hadn't really started my period. A woman is supposed to be fickle, but not her girl parts! The whole period thing was even more frustrating than usual. Then, I realized it was a full moon.

Missed Conception

For those of you who don't believe in the effects a full moon can have, you have not worked in the mental health field. The only thing I can predict during a full moon is my Full Moon Fight with DH.

Right on schedule, he and I had one of our worst fights to date. Normally when we fight, I stay angry for 24 hours or so while I calculate how I can make it work to my advantage. Women should at least get a nice dinner, (preferably a visit to the spa), for compensation of the emotional toll the fight caused. If not, she is not maximizing what she should be getting out of her marriage. Do *not* take marriage advice from me though!

When I am about to do a fertility treatment, and DH and I have a huge fight, the resolution is not as routine as I would like it to be. I begin to question everything. What if we have an argument like that in front of our future child? What if we can't agree on how to raise our future child? What if we should not be having this future child together?

Then things settle down, and I remind myself that as much as I like to plan and schedule, sometimes a little faith provides more stability than any detailed plans could.

So by the time I had begun spotting, had

a fight with DH, and eventually got over the fight, it had been 6 days. I was still just spotting.

I called the doctor's office for the third time to describe my "spotting." At this point, we decided that during previous treatments I had been starting my Clomid on the third day of my spotting; not the third day of my full flow. So the day that I am supposed to start my medication is actually what is usually the last day of my period, because my full flow is only three days. Confused? So was I! Anyway, the phone call ended with the consensus being that this time I would give myself a shot to induce my period if I had not started by Monday.

Less than 24 hours later, I started my period. Three days later, my period stopped, but I began the Femara. At first the Femara seemed fabulous compared to Clomid. Other than sobbing face down in the bed, because I couldn't get the volume button on the remote to work, I felt emotionally in control. I also did not have extreme bloating like on the Clomid.

A few days into the Femara though, I started to notice an excruciating pain in my heels. It was as though I didn't have feet to distribute the weight of a step. If this was God's way of keeping me off my feet, it worked well even into the first week after the IUI.

When I did have to get up . . . and by "have to" I mean to do such things as my neurotic painting of closet doors and the trim in the kitchen, there were a few things I found that provided me relief. First, I sacrificed my cute sandals for tennis shoes or Under Armour's fabulous flip flops which I went out and bought that week. Secondly, I tried Moduko's detox foot pads. (It is amazing the random crap DH finds when he cleans out his top dresser drawer.) Placebo effect or not, the detox pads actually seemed to help. I also rested with ice packs on my heels which also seemed to ease the pain.

Unfortunately detox pads, ice nor anything else could help the other side effect I had: hair loss. After having to use Draino in the tub, because of all the hair I was losing in the shower, I went from washing my hair every day to every third day. About the time I was convinced I would be seeing a bald spot, the hair loss started to slow down.

* * *

When we went in to the doctor's for the ultrasound on a Tuesday, we learned that the side effects had been well worth it. I had two follicles that were "perfect" size at 15 mm.

I have always said that my second IUI would be the one that worked. Leaving the doctor's office that day, I was convinced I was right and hadn't just been telling myself what I wanted to hear.

That Thursday, I gave myself another Ovidrel shot. Again, I did it twice to make sure that I had gotten every last drop.

I hate to think that a husband might read this, and me give away an opportunity for him to be in awe of his wife (he should be anyway), but the Ovidrel shot really does not hurt. This is coming from a woman who is such a big baby that I suck on laughing gas for an hour before the dentist can even lean the chair back. So please, set any anxieties over the Ovidrel shot aside!

As expected, the day before the IUI was filled with anticipation.

8/17/12

Dear Baby,

Psalms 46:10 says, "Be still, and know that I am God." Your great-grandpa would always tell me to "be still" when I was little whether it was when we were in church or if he was trying to get me to go to sleep. I have tried to make "be still" my mantra all day.

Daddy actually took today and even tomorrow off of work. Even though he tried to fill the day with distractions, my mind has been on you. Tomorrow is our 2nd IUI.

I am starting to have nerves over not being a perfect mother. I know there is no such thing, but I wouldn't mind being the first!

We saw an inspiring movie tonight about an infertile couple who were given a little boy with special insights. He told them to never give up trying to have a child. I promise you, we will never give up on having you. Never.

The trophy after a marathon is so much sweeter than one after a sprint. We know every obstacle that we have encountered in having you will bring us only that much greater happiness in the end.

You are worth everything we do. Just the hope of you makes my heart so happy. I am so grateful for hope.

Love,
Mommy

Missed Conception

Steak and Coffee Cake
Chapter 14

I had thought the second IUI would be harder, because I would be able to put even more detail into my anxieties. Surprisingly, my nerves were far calmer this time.

We chose to only tell one of my friends and my brother-in-law when the IUI was scheduled. Despite it usually being impossible for me to keep a secret, I think only having a couple people know the exact date of the IUI, actually did take some of the pressure off of me.

Once we got to the doctor's office, the same crotchety old receptionist made a few miserable comments. Not being quite as hormonal this time, I was able to give it to her that I would probably be the same way if I had to deal with masturbating men all day. Other than that, things went smoothly until the actual IUI.

During this IUI, it felt like the hornet from the previous procedure had unloaded its entire nest inside of me. I am not sure what the deal was, but I am sure that I was stabbed three times, and with that, my timeline begins:

Saturday afternoon: I decided not to get acupuncture this time, as my right index finger seems to still have something going on with the nerve from the last appointment. Instead, I took a four or five hour nap and experienced minimal cramping.

Sunday: I had a mild headache and minimal cramping and twinges.

Monday: I was so tired! I had very vivid dreams and woke up with a migraine. Monday evening I had mild cramping.

Tuesday: My heels were finally starting to feel better. Small clumps of hair had also stopped falling out. I was very tired again, and the vivid dreams continued.

Wednesday: More dreams! I began to look at iPhone apps to see what might be going on in possible fetal development. I was still so tired. Perhaps I was craving chocolate more . . . but with me and chocolate, it is hard to say.

By Wednesday night though, I was eating my third turkey hot dog (at 12:30 at night) when DH pointed out to me that had to be a craving. I didn't think pregnancy cravings started that soon, but I was glad he was helping me justify my midnight snacks! Then I panicked as I Googled turkey hot dogs and realized they had nitrates too. Ugh, nothing is safe to eat!

<u>Thursday:</u> The most pinching and twinges of the past week were experienced. I was very hopeful it was implantation. My sense of smell was noticeably heightened at this point as the smell of my new fabulous boots made me want to return them. Don't worry; I didn't go to such extremes! I was also too tired after shopping for the boots to want to go to another store - absolutely unheard of!

Too much information, as always, but my pee also had smelled so strong this week.

I laid in bed all day with a heating pad on my stomach. I felt like a hen lying on a nest, but that wasn't the first time or the last I would feel like a farm animal during this fertility process.

I also started making my pineapple core smoothies. The U.K. has some alternative suggestions for fertility that I haven't read about on websites from here in the States. One of them was to eat 1/5 of the pineapple core each day for the five days after ovulating. So I started as soon as I read the advice. Mind you, I had to gag it down over the toilet some days, because I don't really care for pineapple to begin with, but I would try anything!

Okay, confessional time. The pineapple sounds healthy and all, but I guess I should come clean with what else was on my grocery list that day. Coffee Cake. Let me give credit where credit is due: Sara Lee's Butter Streusel Coffee Cake to be exact. Yes, I went to the grocery store just to get coffee cake and pineapple.

Although my real rock bottom was on the way back from the grocery store. I had decided to stop at Panera and get myself a Steak Balsamico Sandwich. Unfortunately, it was no longer on the menu. Once a vegetarian for almost 7 years, I found myself walking this poor teenage boy through detailed instructions on how to perfectly meet my cravings for steak. DO NOT forget the add-on of horseradish sauce!

While I'm telling it all, I might as well tell it all. That coffee cake was gone by the next day . . . and I had not shared.

<u>Friday</u>: I still had very vivid dreams, but all other symptoms seemed to have

vanished. Maybe all of this was just side effects of the Ovidrel shot?

Missed Conception

A Long Time in the Making
Chapter 15

8/27/12

Dear Baby,

Last night, I feared the IUI did not work. With prayers and faith, I have reason today to think it was possibly implantation bleeding - you burrowing into my uterus for nine months of bonding that I am so thrilled to experience. We will test on Saturday!

Faith is being sure of what we hope for and certain of what we do not see. Hebrews 11:1.

Love,
Mommy

Well, I definitely did not make it to

Saturday. Come on, who was I kidding? I had never waited until the day I was supposed to test. Trying to be content with hope being enough of a gift got me until Wednesday night. By Thursday, I was at my beloved Target getting a pregnancy test. Luckily for me, it was buy two get one free!

Pregnancy test #1. Realizing that I could be setting myself up for another false positive, I tried to keep my anticipation under control.

When I checked the test, there was a line. A faint line, but a line. I felt all blood drain from my head. I knew that I was pregnant. I knew that this was not just the shot. And then the phone rang.

Throughout the phone call with my mother, I babbled on about random things not wanting to tell her yet. I did tell DH that night though. Having become skeptical of getting hopes up, he remained doubtful. I told him I was 100% sure.

So we agreed that I would test again the following night after he got home from work. If the line was darker, according to my fertility board chat room, I was definitely pregnant.

Twenty minutes after he went to work the next day, I decided I had waited long enough and went ahead and took another test.

Could it be darker?

I loaded the picture on to the IUI support group website I had found. Women from several different states, the U.K. and even Australia immediately began posting their congratulations.

I called the doctor's office and begged to be seen before the long Labor Day weekend. Appointment confirmed.

After DH got home that night, I took the test as we had agreed without mentioning I had already tested. It was even darker than the one in the morning. He looked like he had been caught with his hand in the cookie jar. I then showed him the second one and told him I already had an appointment. Neither of us slept that night.

I was at the doctor's 15 minutes early the next morning which on a Saturday morning is impressive even for neurotic me. The blood was drawn, and now I would need to wait until early afternoon for the results.

But I didn't really need to wait, I already knew.

9/1/12

Dear Baby,
    Well, it's true! You are snuggled

inside of me working hard to grow! Three pregnancy tests, and Daddy and I still couldn't believe it!

The doctor's office called today to report that my blood results confirmed I am pregnant. My Beta (which is the pregnancy hormone) was 146. They wanted at least 100. My progesterone (which supports the pregnancy hormone) was 45. They wanted to see at least 20.

After I hung up, I collapsed in tears of joy. Thank you for making me feel like every day from now on will be like Christmas morning!

My life has forever changed.

Love,
Mommy

Holy Bagoonzas
Chapter 16

The two weeks after our pregnancy was confirmed are a fog. It was so surreal that the concept consumed our minds. We were functioning on no sleep but pure excitement. DH commented on how it was okay that we weren't getting sleep, because parents are supposed to be able to operate without sleep. WRONG. I need my sleep. I desperately need my sleep. So after all family members had been told, (yes, we told family immediately), I went home and finally was able to sleep.

I woke up about a month . . . or two later. Honestly, I don't know how pregnant women who work full-time do it. I fell into a deep love affair with my couch the first couple of months of pregnancy, and I am pretty sure a forklift wouldn't have been able to get me up and at a job by 8 or 9 in the morning. Props to pregnant working women!

A forklift wasn't only needed for getting me off of the couch. My breasts, more commonly referred by me as my bagoonzas, needed a forklift, not a bra. As I was standing in the living room talking to DH one evening, I heard a snap. My underwire had snapped under the weight of my ever growing chest.

Not only were they huge, but they were sore. Cover your bagoonzas before turning around in the shower to wash your face, or you may have your nips violated by the stream of water in ways you have never wanted.

Not only were my bagoonzas huge, but my stomach was growing quickly. I thought that when I was pregnant my always large and in charge stomach wouldn't be judged. Oh how I was wrong. People love asking how far along you are and then blatantly staring at your belly with that judgmental big eyeball gaze. You have to love when someone thinks it's acceptable to say, "Are you *sure* there's only one baby in there, and you are not having at least twins?"

However, pregnant women have a fabulous secret they keep from the rest of the world. Maternity pants. They are genius! They are the most comfortable clothes a person could wear. I recommend all women buying a pair just so that you don't have to do the sneaky unbutton-the-jeans-under-the-dinner-table move. Maternity jeans never betray you!

When I walked into the pregnancy boutique at only five weeks, I felt like someone was going to yell "imposter!" It still seemed too good to be true that I was finally pregnant. That didn't stop me from buying two pairs of jeans, Burt's Bees all-natural Belly Butter and Preggie Pops. The sales associate even put a pacifier sample in the bag. I was loving every cute part of this pregnancy thing!

* * *

DH and I had our first pregnancy ultrasound. I realized I had been holding my breath when the doctor announced that everything looked fine. There was no ectopic pregnancy. There was not an empty egg sack. This wasn't a false pregnancy. This was not any of the nightmares that my internet searches had told me about. This was really happening, but exactly when it was going to happen, we still didn't know. I had been too overwhelmed to remember to get the due date confirmed!

When we got home from the doctor's, DH hung the ultrasound picture on the bedroom wall. I immediately began assembling a stroller / car seat system that I had ordered a few days after the positive pregnancy test. What pregnant woman can resist a baby sale at Target?

* * *

By 7 ½ weeks, I was back again at the maternity boutique. The doctor had explained at our visit that some women who have done fertility, begin to show early like women who have had previous pregnancies. I think he was just being nice. In my defense though, despite the growing belly, I had lost 4 pounds since finding out that I was pregnant. A few food aversions and some Metformin side effects contributed to this weight loss. Whatever the cause of the weight loss, as DH so eloquently put it, "You'd never be able to tell."

This time at the maternity clothes shop, I bought enough pieces for a basic wardrobe that I was hoping would get me through a significant part of the pregnancy. I hate that discounted maternity clothes are not as available as discounted regular clothing. I also hate that whoever is designing maternity clothing thinks that I like ridiculously flashy colors and crazy patterns. At least we have evolved past the muu muu.

Then I tried on the bras. I usually am a 36DD, and by "usually" I mean since seventh grade. So, I gave a 40E a try. The 40 part was too big and the E was far too small. I was advised that there was a bra boutique for women "with my situation" on the North side of town. Bras are expensive, and I am not the best at finding random places in a different part of town. So, I decided to "weight" it out. Surely this rampant growth spurt would slow down?

Missed Conception

Too Good to be True?
Chapter 17

While pregnant, most people bombarded me with excitement. Most of the time, this was incredible to experience and made me realize how loved by so many my baby would be. Although, sometimes it was overwhelming, and I would find myself not able to match the other person's excitement. I then came to the realization that for the most part, this pregnancy just seemed too good to be true.

Of course there were changes going on with my body, so on some level I realized I really was pregnant. But to be honest, if it had not been for the ultrasounds, I would not have been able to believe I was pregnant. It was just so surreal. How do you want something your entire life, and in such a short time be able to process that you have finally received that gift?

Missed Conception

At 8 weeks, I went to the bathroom and noticed some brown blood on the toilet paper. This could not be happening. Was this pregnancy truly going to be too good to be true? Was this baby already being taken away from me? I had been so sure that our obstacles were a thing of the past, and we had jumped our last hurdle when we received the positive pregnancy test.

The fertility office reassured me that brown blood was old blood, and if it did not progress, there was nothing to worry about. The internet told me all blood was considered a "threatened miscarriage." I kept going back to the bathroom to check, but it seemed to be going away.

A few days later we had another appointment with the fertility specialist. He reassured me that spotting would be normal during the first trimester. We then had another ultrasound, and there was our baby. Not a gray spot on the monitor, but a tiny being with arms, legs, a belly, and a very big head. The baby was also suspended upside down. We were already able to see the spine and even hear the heartbeat! *Wow*, we were having a baby!

At a complete loss for words, I hugged

the doctor while wearing my paper towel gown. Through tears, I uttered, "Thanks for making my life."

As I walked out of the fertility office, a very unexpected wariness and even sadness came over me. This was the office that I had initially so resented having to enter. This was also the office though that had held my hand, given me hope, walked me through my frustrations, and understood what I had been through. Sometimes, I had come here as often as a few times a week. Over time, I had learned to have trust that this staff would be the ones to make my baby possible. They were always only a phone call away. They knew my body. They were even there when my baby was conceived! This doctor's office had become an extension of my family, and now I was going to have to trust another office to get me through the remainder of the nine months.

* * *

Once able to detect a fetal heartbeat, the chance of miscarriage is very similar to that at the end of the first trimester. DH and I decided that even though it was earlier than most people chose, we wanted to share our news with our friends. Knowing there was still a chance of miscarriage, I reminded myself no pregnancy was guaranteed at any point throughout the pregnancy. I had waited long enough to experience this, and I wanted to share what I was experiencing. No more secrets.

Telling our friends made the pregnancy so real. It was also so freeing to be able to openly talk about our pregnancy.

There were reactions however that I had not expected. A few women told me throughout the pregnancy that they were just so jealous of me. When this happened, it was always such a reality shock that I had become "that woman" I had always envied. I was the one having the baby. I would always earnestly reassure them that they too would be amazing moms someday. Their jealousy not only flooded me with appreciation and peace over being pregnant, but also grounded me with the reminder that this pregnancy truly was such a gift. A gift unfortunately not every deserving woman will receive.

Another reaction that I experienced from others was judgment. Shockingly, people responded with questioning my understanding of the possibility that I could miscarry. Some even whispered stories of their own miscarriage to others around me.

As though people's whispers or perhaps my confidence in telling people early somehow jinxed us, we had a scare. Quite a scare.

I had just received an app alert on my phone that I was 10 weeks pregnant. As I was announcing the details of the baby's growth to my husband (yes, while I was peeing), I looked down and saw bright red blood. There was a significant amount on the toilet paper as though I had started my period. I felt lightheaded and began to panic. I knew the blood being red was far more of a concern.

My panicking actually prevented me from even remembering how to use my phone for a minute. Once my fingers remembered how to dial, I first called the midwife's office that we had an appointment to meet. They didn't want to see me since I had not had my initial visit. I then called my primary doctor who was right down the road. His receptionist simply said to get to the emergency room. My fertility doctor had specifically told me not to rush off to the emergency room at the sight of spotting. This seemed a little more than spotting, but I decided to call the fertility office to see if their opinion would remain the same.

The fertility office called me back 45 excruciating minutes later. Again, they assured me that spotting was normal. While waiting for the phone call, the bleeding at least had not gotten worse. Even with minor cramping, they told me to rest and try to be calm. I moved as little as possible, but I was absolutely not calm.

In fact, this last episode of spotting made me check the toilet paper throughout the rest of my pregnancy. I felt like I'd had no control over my body when I was trying to get pregnant since there was no simply willing it to cooperate. Now, I realized that I did have some control in the fertility process. It was after becoming pregnant, that beyond reasonable means, I realized I was not in control. It was almost a strange, unfamiliar sense of entrapment. I was pregnant for the day, but after such a scare, I did not know what the next day would bring. This would be a frightening, long pregnancy if I couldn't overcome this anxiety.

* * *

A little over a week after the last episode of spotting, we had our first appointment with the midwives' office. The midwife held the Doppler device to my stomach to hear the heartbeat. There was no heartbeat.

Not hearing a heartbeat at this appointment had been my greatest fear since spotting. I could sense DH tensing up and sitting very still next to me. I could not look over at him. How had I been so sure this pregnancy would be fine and yet have it end so soon? I just stared at the magazine rack on the wall.

The midwife assured us that it might just be too early to use the Doppler on the stomach and went to go speak to the ultrasound tech for more accurate testing. I still could not look over at DH. He was literally radiating worry, and the look on his face would solidify my fear.

We moved to the ultrasound room, and within seconds of the ultrasound, the baby's heartbeat was detected. Everything was fine. The midwife announced that our baby needed a spanking after that scare. Hm. No, the midwife needed to learn when to use certain machines, and I needed a Xanax! (No, pregger me did not really take a Xanax!)

That scare over, along with my first trimester, the midwife now wanted me to go off of my Metformin. She also wanted me to be screened early for gestational diabetes. I was beginning to learn the complications from PCOS do not end with conception.

I was also learning that my insurance pretty much covered nothing. Now that I was at a midwife's office, everything was maternity related and could not be billed as PCOS related. Nothing was covered. On top of that, I failed my first sugar test.

I do not do well with failing any test, let alone, one that I have to fast for. Twelve hours without food and four vials of blood later, the second test was complete. I was in line for McDonald's french fries (don't judge), and results had confirmed I did not have diabetes.

10/23/12

Dear Baby,

You are growing so fast, (about the size of my pinky), yet it is still so hard to believe my little miracle is on its way!

We have had a few scares since I last wrote, but the Dr. assures me you are fine. We have now had three ultrasounds where we have seen your constant growth. Your heartbeat last time was 166. Old wives' tales say that means you are a girl. I'm amazed that I have no intuition yet as to what you are going to be. Your Nanny swears you are a girl.

Morning sickness still hasn't been too bad. I've only thrown up 3-4 times, but my food aversions are awful. I cried for 20 minutes the other night, because Daddy brought home wings to eat during a football game. The thought of meat or the smell of barbeque or hot sauce is AWFUL! I've lost 8lbs and have started drinking protein shakes, but hopefully meat will soon sound good to me.

My belly is growing every day, and I think it is really starting to dawn on Daddy this is happening. He has been so helpful lately.

I am almost finished switching my closet over to get everything out of your room. Nanny and I are going to go open a registry weekend after next to celebrate being finished with my first trimester. I am so excited for this - to finally be the one who gets to pick out all the cute things for my own baby! Keep growing little one!

Love,
Mommy

Pinnacle of Cynical
Chapter 18

With all of the scares, and the exhaustion, I was really feeling frustrated. Yes, I wanted this pregnancy – the good, the bad, and the ugly moments of it. That doesn't mean I am not human, and it certainly doesn't mean I do not have hormones!

The first trimester was complete! I celebrated by registering at Babies R Us. It was surreal knowing I was actually registering for *my* baby shower. (If "surreal" is starting to be repetitious, it's because there really is no way else to explain how I felt during pregnancy.)

Unfortunately, registering was only one afternoon; a small blip of a nine month period. Everyone had told me that I would feel great by the second trimester. Why did I not feel great?

"If I had a sister," was a phrase that ran

through my head a lot during this time. If I had a sister, I would have learned how to apply eyeliner a lot earlier in life. I was beginning to realize there are a lot of other things I would have expected her to have filled me in on too.

Perhaps a sister would have informed me that I would grow mass peach fuzz on my stomach when I was pregnant. That the CONSTANT peeing would start immediately. That the insomnia can also start immediately. Ligament pain is sharp and can set in early on in pregnancy. Maybe a sister could have answered how I was supposed to stay on top of my dental hygiene when I would throw up every time I brushed my teeth! A sister would have also maybe told me that applying for a job while pregnant is a joke; no, common sense should have filled me in on that one. For all those times I had said I would never eat anything unhealthy while I was pregnant, a sister would have laughed at me and set me straight.

It is not that *everything* I ate was unhealthy, but food aversions are morning sickness's partner in crime that I had never heard discussed. "Food aversions" is just not a violent enough term to fully describe how vulgar some foods can be to a pregnant woman. It's as though the aroma/stench of these foods is being poured down your nose and throat in some kind of water-boarding torture saga. As much as I tried to will myself to eat healthy, vegetables were repulsive. Chicken was even more offensive. Hot sauce and barbeque sauce were the worst.

Unfortunately, DH's sympathy cravings consisted of wings, wings, and more wings. One night he walked through the front door with a carry- out of wings. I locked myself in the bedroom and sobbed. Food smells violated my life.

With such strong food aversions, I was 4 ½ months pregnant and was still losing weight. After going through fertility treatments and the exhaustion and nausea from the first four months of pregnancy, I felt like I had been pregnant for years. Going off of the Metformin seemed not to have made any difference in how I felt.

When I did feel like eating, the restrictions were numerous. No lunch meat, no soft cheeses, no lobster, no hollandaise. One time I gave in and had a turkey sandwich. I then had "Listeria hysteria" and convinced myself I had done irreversible damage to the baby. The midwife assured me I had not, but she did stress the importance of having more protein. So, I comforted myself with a protein shake here and there and stuck to just eating what sounded good to me.

1/15/12

Dear Baby,

We had another doctor appointment today. You are now big enough we can hear your heartbeat from the Doppler machine on my belly: 160 beats/minute. December 11th is when I will find out if you are a boy or a girl. I can not wait!

I went to a breastfeeding meeting. It was pretty intense and lots of serious hippies. I am really nervous about the breastfeeding - the lack of schedule, the pain, how it leaves your dad out. I know it's so much healthier for you though, and it's free. Another breastfeeding group I went to seemed much less intimidating, and the women served as proof it can be done!

I am really showing. My energy is slowly coming back, but food is still often really gross. Orange juice, bananas, milk and McDonald's french fries are about the only things that consistently sound good. I really hope healthy foods start sounding good again soon!

I announced on Facebook today my pregnancy. So many people are excited for your arrival. You are already so loved!

It is really starting to sink in that I am pregnant. I think I felt you on Tuesday when Daddy and I were driving to get our flu shots. A little tickle a couple inches below my belly button. You are always right on my bladder.

Love, Love, Love,
Mommy

Missed Conception

If I were Ann Landers . . .
Chapter 19

Even though pregnancy had its rough patches, there were several positive things about being pregnant that resulted in new experiences and feelings. If I were Ann Landers, my advice would be to be your own heroine in harrowing times. Make pregnancy work for you!

As I had suspected when struggling with fertility, people are nicer to pregnant women! When you're not pregnant, this is so unfair. When you are pregnant, it's over the top, but it's nice. Initially, I felt guilty receiving people's abundant concern and kindness just because I was pregnant. I wasn't handicapped, I was pregnant. Then I realized that this was the support I would have liked while doing fertility, and that this was the support I'd probably be wishing I had in the future when I was at home with a sick toddler puking all over me when I myself was sick. The point is, enjoy it. Whether you feel you deserve the reason for the kindness, you deserve the kindness.

One example of this random kindness was the man in the grocery store parking lot who approached me and offered to walk the cart back for me. Yes, I could have easily done it myself. But it was cold, and it was a nice gesture, and it was awesome. He might have just been a super nice guy; however, chivalry is pretty much dead, and although it can be resuscitated every now and then, I'm pretty sure he did that for me because I was pregnant.

So indulge in other's kindness, and also use your pregnancy experience as an opportunity to soften your own heart. Going through infertility makes you tough. You have to thicken your skin, brace yourself for disappointment, and learn to move on. Being pregnant reminds you that it's okay to be a sap. It's okay to revel and enjoy this pregnancy, all fears aside. I tried so hard to soak in every minute of this pregnancy. I knew it might be the only time I ever experienced a baby inside of me, and I didn't want to take one moment for granted.

Part of soaking in every moment of the pregnancy is learning to embrace your pregnant body. Around five months pregnant, I went to Great Clips to get a haircut. During the haircut, I passed out. This could have been divine intervention, trying to prevent me from a bad haircut, but really it was my body telling me to pay attention. For once in my life, I needed to eat more.

Our entire lives, women are bombarded with pressure to be thin, and this doesn't end when you're pregnant. Try being pregnant the same time as Kate Middleton! I never tried to be on a diet while I was pregnant, but I was worried about gaining weight. Passing out made me realize, I needed to stop being confined by the restraints I've always been under as a female and instead, eat what sounded good when it sounded good. My body was telling me how to nourish this baby, and I needed to listen.

By 5 ½ months, I had gained 6lbs. I'd started out overweight, so I didn't need to gain as much as the average person. My body was definitely getting bigger though, which was exciting because it meant my baby was getting bigger!

Not only was my belly growing, but my

body was changing in lots of other ways. All of those changes that can be intimidating and overwhelming should try to be seen as ways nature will surprise you with how it can prepare for your baby. Since it was hard to have that insight, I tried to at least have a little humor.

I woke up one morning to discover that I had drooled. DH pointed out to me that I couldn't have drooled that far off my pillow. Then what on Earth was that? Hm . . . yep, I had nipple leakage. It was exciting that my boobs were working as they needed to, but freaky as hell, my friends.

Not only did I have leakage from new places, but then there was the hair issue. The luscious locks are all over. You might as well find it funny that your entire pregnant body pretty much morphs into a Chia Pet owned by an intoxicated Edward Scissorhands. You just can't see what you're shaving. If you can see it, chances are you can't reach it.

You are not always going to have a glowing aura surrounding you. There are gross things about pregnancy, but what your body is doing is amazing and you should take pride in knowing day by day you are being changed inside and out.

Katherine Shields

For these changes, you should be rewarded. So indulge. There is fun in pregnancy. Design the nursery. Even if you're not crafty, do some DIY nursery projects. My baby won't care I can't sew.

My favorite indulgence is always a massage. Massages are indulgent but very practical too! Now is the time to treat yourself like a princess – before your little prince or princess steals your throne!

Missed Conception

It's a . . .
Chapter 20

Are you craving sweet or salty? Are you carrying low or high? What month did you conceive? Let's do the "Pencil Test." Let's look at the Chinese calendar. Let's buy a gender test. Let's plan the nursery down to every possible detail and argue over every possible name of both genders. The excitement, anticipation, and frivolous planning leading up to finding out the gender of your baby just prepares you for the reality that no matter how much you prepare, you are often left totally without control.

I don't know how women who wait until they deliver to find out the gender do it. Lots of people suggested I wait, because "there's no better surprise." I'm pretty sure it is a surprise whether I find out at four months or nine months. I'm also pretty sure that a baby coming out of my vagina is a big enough surprise for one day.

Missed Conception

Our ultrasound tech was about as pleasant as a rock in your shoe. It was the end of the day, and she obviously could not care less what the gender of our baby was. I on the other hand, was so anxious I felt like I was going to get sick as I walked down the hall to the examining room. Then, I looked over at the board full of birth announcements hanging in the hallway, and say what you will, but suddenly I just knew I was going to have a little girl. So far, I had been convinced I was having a boy, but my intuition had instantly flipped.

As we entered the room, the tech informed me that "most women were anxious over health, not gender." She then asked if something was "wrong," since I was having my ultrasound at 18 weeks instead of 20 weeks. Something was going to be wrong if this woman didn't pop a Prozac, slap a smile on her face and act like this was the most exciting moment of her life too!

Miss kill-joy projected the ultrasound on the wall, and informed us in her monotone voice, something about the baby's nose bone indicating that it was not Down Syndrome. She then pointed out all 4 chambers of the heart . . . I hadn't even thought to worry about each chamber of the heart! Wonder what else I hadn't thought to worry about that I should be?

The jolly tech continued, "Oh, and it looks like it's a girl, and here is the hand, and she's moving a lot. Did you have caffeine?"

WHAT? The tech had just announced I was going to have a daughter the way Ben Stein talks about "dry eyes" during a Visine commercial!

Up on my elbows, I urged, "Are you sure it's a girl? Like, I can go buy pink paint, dresses, and tell everyone I know, sure?"

Miss personality just said, "We're not allowed to say 100%, so let's say 98%."

As we were leaving the appointment, DH looked over again at the board of birth announcements and said, "What about the name Olivia?" Now, I had suggested this name several times before, but I'm such a slow learner when it comes to letting a man think ideas are his . . . except for this time. Not only did we know the gender, but we now had a name.

The day was not over though. We needed to go to the mall. I was on a mission for girl clothing, and I think poor DH just needed a chair to sit down and take it all in. This daughter was already more expensive than a son would be . . . and well worth every penny!

12/20/12

Dear Baby,

Well, the articles that I read say you can hear now. I'm sorry you have to listen to me sing along to the radio!

I just took my first bath since being pregnant. They say warm ones are great, but hot ones are dangerous. I've been too nervous to not do everything by the book, but boy was it relaxing.

Since being pregnant, I've also started eating hamburgers for the first time in 12 years. I was a vegetarian for a very long time, and red meat is usually still so gross. Actually, all meat while pregnant has been gross. Pork is always a no. Did you know pigs have the mental capacity of a 3-year-old? Daddy says he won't feed you hot dogs from pork - tell on him if he does!

My pregnancy cravings seem to be: popcorn, granola bars, juice,

Hershey kisses, fruit, McDonald's french fries with lots of ketch-up, Mac n Cheese, pizza and french onion soup. I swear I'm much healthier of an eater when not pregnant. I used to always say I wouldn't put anything unhealthy in my mouth when I was pregnant. I'd be starving you if I followed that rule! I can finally stand to eat salads again, and most days have more energy. Still no weight gain, but you are growing fine, and I look VERY pregnant.

We had our ultrasound Dec. 18th. You measured exactly perfect at 18 weeks, and 3 days. You weighed 8 ½ ounces and are in the 43rd percentile. We got to see you go from all scrunched up to a big stretch. What an amazing early Christmas gift! Then we were told - you are a girl! Look out world, a princess is on her way!

Love,
Mommy

Missed Conception

Mind Race to the Finish
Chapter 21

I was thrilled to know what the gender of my baby was going to be. Details always make a dream more of a reality. Pure emotion of any type is often quickly muddled with other factors though – especially when you are a hormone raging woman!

Defining my baby by gender was an incredibly exciting part in the adventure to welcoming her into this world. Perfectly coinciding with this new level of excitement was the realization that I was not having a son. I'm assuming any mother might experience this mix of emotions to an extent, but it seemed a little more defined for me having gone through fertility.

When I first found out I was pregnant, there was a part of me that really wanted twins in order to guarantee that I would be the mother to more than one child. After finding out I was pregnant with a singleton, the realization that this was probably my only child was totally masked by the incredible elation that I was at least having a child. After finding out the baby was a girl, that realization crept back in coming to terms with the real possibility that I probably wouldn't ever be pregnant again nor have the chance to have a son.

I know this chapter makes me sound like an ingrate. Confessing my realization that I wouldn't have a mama's boy, and worrying that my husband was at peace with not having a son, by no means is to convey I was not so happy to be having a little girl. I truly was ecstatic. I just think that the realization this could be my only child was a new wave of closure with infertility.

As often we women do, a thought accompanied with guilt for that thought just exacerbates the emotion. I knew one baby should be more than "enough." It was working through this feeling and not pushing it aside, that led me to the beginning of being so overwhelmingly grateful that I did have a baby to raise. That in-the-moment appreciation prepared me for everything from the uncomfortable moments of labor to the oh-so - sweet and the oh-so-exhausting moments of motherhood.

No matter how hard or wonderful a moment is, that may be the only time I'll have that experience. I want to also always remember that these pregnancy and parenting moments are those that so many women still desperately desire to experience.

Being content was a good lesson to learn since I was already being asked when I was going to have the next baby! To always appreciate and enjoy this miracle, I feel I must always keep it fresh in my mind the hurdles we had to jump to get here. I never want to be desensitized to the pain of infertility. My heart still goes out to, and prayers are still said, for those women I know who deserve a baby just as much as I but have yet to become pregnant.

* * *

Heavy thoughts continued to weigh on my mind. As wonderful as it was to have the problem of worrying about my future child, it still was quite a worry!

Dads often joke they need a shotgun for

the worries that having a girl will bring. Little is said about the worry that a mother of a daughter encounters. As much as I've always wanted a daughter, I don't want her to struggle with her confidence or her weight. I don't want her to have PCOS. I don't want her to have heartbreaks. What if I don't have it all figured out and can't protect her from these things?

Having all those bubbling thoughts lead me to become hyper-aware of the women who surrounded me. I have always been upheld by strong, supportive, intelligent, dynamic women. These women will be the women that surround my daughter as well. My daughter's success as a woman will not rely solely on me, but she will be able to glean examples from all of the strong women I introduce into her life. It sure helps to take the pressure off of me!

Speaking of all those amazing women, they threw me two fabulous baby showers. Sitting at the baby showers, seeing so many people who were so happy for me and so incredibly generous made me feel like the luckiest woman in the world. Clean up the wrapping paper and ribbon, and in front of me was a nursery that others had provided.

After the wrapping paper and ribbon

was indeed cleaned up, everything was taken home to our living room. DH walked in the front door after yet another day of golf, and the look on his face was priceless. "It looks like the Pepto-bismol factory exploded in here!" Yes, when friends and family hear, "it's a girl," EVERYTHING is pink.

Pregnancy isn't all parties though, it does require some serious planning . . . especially for someone like me!

Missed Conception

Neurotic Hypnotic
Chapter 22

A year or so ago, we were in Key West, and I wanted to go snorkeling. I had been snorkeling around a bay before, and I'm a good swimmer. However, I hadn't read the fine print which stated we would be traveling seven miles off shore and jumping off the boat. Even when we zipped up the wet suit and went to jump off the boat, I still thought this was a good idea. Then out of nowhere, I was blindsided with a panic attack. Here I was in the ocean, treading water, nothing to hold on to except the pink kiddie pool noodle later thrown to me. I was having an absolutely cannot breathe panic attack.

If a fun activity on vacation could leave me panic stricken, childbirth easily could. I knew that trillions of women all around the world had gone through labor. Hell, in high school we even read some book about a woman giving birth and then going back out to work in the field. (By the way, to deter high school pregnancies, students probably should not read something that makes labor sound so blasé.) Anyway, knowing other women have done it did not alleviate my fear of having a panic attack during delivery.

I knew this baby was coming out one way or another. But if I panicked while snorkeling, I was sure to panic when an 8 pound freight train came barreling through my vaj.

So being the neurotic, proactive person I am, I began to research childbirth classes. Out of all that were offered, most were a couple hours long or even a full day. Then I spotted it: one claiming to reduce anxiety, and it was a 10-week course. I roped DH in, signed us up, and brought a pink notebook along.

So the breastfeeding class we had gone to was save-a-treeish. This birth-class could save a rainforest. We were to alleviate pain from labor through hypnobirthing – putting ourselves into a hypnotic trance while trusting our body was designed to push another human being out of your hoo-ha.

Wasting no time, the instructor had us

lie on the ground with our partner and listen to the hypnobirthing CD. Neurotic me, could not lie on the ground like everyone else, so I sat. As I sat, I noticed that DH had a whistling booger, there was a wrinkle in my sock, the guy next to me smelled like cigarettes, I still needed to clean the dishes when I got home, and I needed to call about adding the baby to my health insurance. DH was asleep by the time the CD ended, and I had chewed off all my nails. Well, at least one of us would make it through childbirth.

Throughout the weeks of childbirth, the idea was consistently brought up that an epidural was not necessary. The theory is that medical interventions, in general, shouldn't be seen as mandatory for a natural bodily function. Despite Western modernization and practice, a natural bodily function is exactly what childbirth is.

I had never considered giving birth without an epidural. I had a spinal tap done once, though, and hated being so out of control. I was also prone to migraines which epidurals made even riskier. The bug had been put in my ear.

DH kept saying he thought I could bypass the epidural. At first I felt pressured and even more panicked. I had hoped I would go to this childbirth class to hear that the hospital would give me any drug I need and receive a master spreadsheet of what I should pack. Instead, I was gathering all kinds of information of how to best empower me as a mother and as a hospital patient. In addition to that, the thought dawned on me that I could be further empowered by denying the epidural.

Full disclosure clause: I am in 100% agreement with medical intervention when intervention is necessary. I am also a believer in pain medication when physically or mentally necessary. With all that out of the way, for me personally, having a natural childbirth became my way to restore confidence in my body.

While going through fertility, I really struggled with my femininity and confidence in my body. I could not naturally do what so many other women could. Giving birth without any intervention would help instill the confidence in me again to trust my body. And so the plan was formed:

<u>Birth Vision</u>

First stage of Labor:

- Father is to be present at all times during

labor and birth.

- I would like to labor at home as long as possible and request permission to return home should I arrive less than 5cm.
- I would like to have a birthing ball and bathtub.
- If IV is deemed necessary, I would like to have a saline lock so that I may move around as freely as possible. If this becomes too uncomfortable, I'd like to have it removed.
- Please, no internal fetal monitoring, unless emergency arises and with consent.
- Vaginal exams only upon consent, and as few as possible to avoid membrane disruption.
- Please, no Pitocin or breaking of water unless deemed medically necessary.
- No analgesia or anesthesia unless requested. **Please, do not offer!**
- Freedom to move and walk during labor.

Second Stage of Labor:

- Choice of position for pushing.
- We are planning on doing self-directed pushing.

- No episiotomy, please.
- Keep lights low.
- If delivery assistance is needed, please use suction instead of forceps.
- Father would like to catch the baby.
- Please place baby on mother's abdomen, unless medical intervention is necessary.
- Cord to be cut by father, approximately 5 minutes after birth.
- Breastfeed immediately to help birth placenta – no Pitocin, uterine massage, or pulling of cord.
- If stitching is necessary, please use local anesthetic.

Third Stage of Labor:

- Newborn to stay with parents at all times. No nursery visits.
- Please delay all routine exams for at least 2 hours to allow for breastfeeding and bonding time.
- Please perform all physical exams and procedures in room with parents.
- Baby is not to be given the HEP B vaccine.
- If warming is needed, please place on mother's chest with blankets.

- Breastfeeding only: No bottles, pacifiers, artificial nipples, formula or water.
- Father to stay with baby and mother at all times.

*In the event of a C-Section, I would like the father to be present. Unless cause of medical necessity, please allow for baby to remain with parents at all times.

Missed Conception

Nesting and Resting
Chapter 23

Even with birth classes and baby showers, there is a part of you as a woman who still cannot possibly truly absorb how your life has changed and will only continue to change. At 23 weeks, even after having had the gender ultrasound, I still really couldn't grasp that I was pregnant. Then I began to feel her kick. The little kicks and hiccups, and even the rib jabs, served as reminders throughout the remainder of the nine months that this miracle really was happening to me.

I felt so lucky throughout my pregnancy, that when I hit the half-way mark I was the slightest bit melancholy. As silly as it may sound, a small fraction of my daughter's life had already passed. Her short time protected inside of me was coming to an end.

So, I did what any hormonal woman would do, and I sobbed on the couch about how we would not be financially helping her if she chose to go to a college too far away.

Eventually, I got a grip and set my mind to nesting. In addition to the birth classes, I had the epiphany that all paint needed touching up and absolutely no baseboards could be dusty upon the arrival of my Little Miss.

In the midst of my paint-the-kitchen-ceiling escapade, I ended up triggering early contractions. Having never experienced back contractions before, ignorance was bliss and prevented me from panicking too much. I had learned my lesson, though.

I had also learned that early contractions can be caused when your body is out of alignment and the baby is wedged too far back in between your hip and spine. In other words, my extreme nesting had helped position the baby in a way that was pinching my Sciatic Nerve to the point of practically having to crawl in the middle of the night to the bathroom.

Out of desperation, I tried a chiropractor. He was every bit the quack that I had stereotyped a chiropractor to be. That man seriously thought a few taps on the back was going to solve this problem?

Out of even further desperation, I tried another chiropractor. Wow, am I now a believer. Finding a good, well recommended chiropractor whom specializes in maternity, was not easy, but was so worth the search!

What is also so worth it, are prenatal massages. Actually, massages in general are always worth it. They're expensive though, (although I do believe tax deductible), but when you're growing another human being inside you, can you really put a price on your well-being . . . and sanity?

You do definitely question your sanity at times as a pregnant woman: the hormones and the super sense of smell and the peeing of one's pants. Yep, I said it.

DH had got a pastry from the restaurant where we were, and as he looked the other way to pull out from the parking spot, I took a bite - a mammoth bite. What pregnant woman can resist a cheese danish?!

Well, my impromptu devouring of DH's dessert came as a shock to him for some reason. The surprised look on his face got me to laughing . . . and laughing . . . and oh my gosh, MY WATER WAS BREAKING! Or wait, was I peeing my pants? I WAS PEEING MY

PANTS!

If DH was shocked to see most of his danish missing, he sure as shit was shocked to realize I was peeing my pants all over his car seat. He tried shoving a gym shirt from the back seat under my pregnant ass, and I tried kegeling the situation in to control, but the reality was peeing your pants is cool.

At the midwife appointment the following day, I tried to play it off like my water had broken. This only led to being told, "As humbling as it may be, you just peed your pants." Fantastic.

Waiting…Waiting… Anticipating
Chapter 24

4/18/2013

Dar Baby,

So many heightened emotions! Your Grandpa is very, very sick and won't be on this earth much longer. When the doctor told Grandpa last week he had two weeks to live, he explained that he was probably going to need closer to a month, depending on when you chose to make your arrival. Since hearing that, I have been even more certain you would know to come early.

Tuesday, we visited the hospital. The nurse and room were very nice. I want a non-medicated birth- for you, for breastfeeding and to help restore the confidence in my body I lost through fertility treatments. I'm going to do my best for us. I do have such faith in you already and feel you have worked with me so amazingly every step of the way. You have already been an amazing baby!

I was 1 cm dilated on Tuesday. I lost my plug today, (ew, I know), and have had more contractions. I'm guessing you will be here in the next few days. I'm so ready for this crazy, amazing adventure, and I'm so excited to meet you. I am sad to know that my days of feeling you kick and move in my belly are so numbered. I know you will grow up so fast, and I just want to do my best at giving you everything you need.

We're leaning from "Olivia Faye" more towards "Olivia Beatrice." Beatrice means "blessed" and "bringer of joy." It was also your grandpa's mother's name. I could NEVER have guessed what pressure *naming you would be, but "Olivia" is a symbol of peace which you most certainly will bring to this family.*

I love you and am ready to go on this journey with you. SO many people are eager for your arrival. You will truly bring so much peace and joy to this world.

Love,
Mommy

I had been convinced my entire pregnancy that Olivia would be born April 28th. Don't ask why. It was just one of those gut instincts. April 17th, I lost my mucus plug. DH made the mistake of asking what it looked like – "a kidney bean, covered in a hocker." Yep, it's just as gross as it sounds folks. According to my WebMD degree, losing the mucous plug meant I should have the baby in about a week.

First thing is first: my birthday, April 19th. My dad's health had rapidly declined in the past couple weeks, so we decided to spend the day with my parents and brother who was in town. I pulled a chair next to my dad in hopes that he would get to feel the baby kick. I also told him we had decided on the name

"Olivia Beatrice." Beatrice was my dad's mother, and by the look on his face, he was a huge fan of the name. We had a great visit, and I even busted out my belly to show how my belly-button now popped in and out with each breath, just to get a laugh or two. When saying goodbye, my dad was delighted to be able to finally address my stomach with a name.

Two weeks had passed and no baby. I really couldn't wrap my head around how I was still physically carrying this baby. The heat, even though it was only May, was unbearable. My feet had begun to swell too.

Sidenote: Deafen yourself to others' stories. I began to learn that like a fisherman's tales, women's pregnancy stories become even more impressive with time. I don't care if you were playing softball 40 weeks pregnant. My ass was on the couch with the air conditioner on 66. I felt like her head was going to literally fall out every time I stood up. Gross? Well, things get a lot more descriptive . . . .

Anyway, three weeks later, my due date had arrived, and still no baby. I attempted to do yard work to again try to get labor started. It ended up with me just dumping the plant on the dirt and walking away.

The other yard news, was that my crazy,

literally bat-shit crazy, neighbor was in my yard with a chain saw chopping down my bushes as my mother called to tell me my dad (who was now in the nursing home) was struggling to live through the day. If all of that wasn't going to send me in to labor, nothing would.

The following day was Mother's Day. I had been certain since finding out I was pregnant, that this Mother's Day would be MY day. I obviously hadn't learned, even with all the fertility, that God's schedule is much different than mine. Not only had I not had my baby April 28th, but I most certainly was still pregnant May 12th. No baby, meant DH still thought the day was all about my Mother-in-Law which included her expecting us all to be at a barbeque restaurant; yes, barbeque, the most offensive of smells to pregnant me . . . . I wonder if she was well aware of that.

Before going to dinner, we made the drive to Indiana to visit my dad in the nursing home. It obviously wasn't the Mother's Day my mom would have planned either. It was so frustrating having to wait until DH's days off to go to Indiana, but traveling out of state in the last month didn't seem like a good idea. I guess this was one of God's ways of teaching me all things must come second to my child.

There was my dad's name on the little slip next to the door of his room in the nursing home. What a difference from the name plate on his office desk where I'm sure he was so yearning to be sitting. The name of your parent next to a nursing home room is something nobody wants to ever see. My dad, the strong, brilliant attorney, was now in a wheelchair struggling to mentally connect the dots of what was all happening around him.

Oh how my dad's face lit up though when we walked through the door. For that split second, it was like I had my dad back. Most of the visit, however, was conversations that didn't make sense and him being very frustrated with being in a wheelchair.

As we went to leave, I had DH take a picture of my dad touching my belly. As he did, he told me, "You know, she's just not quite ready to come yet. She needs a few more days." Then he chuckled and told me, "She's going to look Chinese." Thinking that he was again struggling to stay mentally focused, I gave him a hug and kiss and said goodbye.

As I walked the long hallway back to the car, my eyes stung with the tears that told me what I had already known for a week or so.

Even if my dad could just hold on a few more days for me to have this baby, it wouldn't be the same.

5/12/13

Dear Baby,

I am still pregnant! You must take after your daddy - being late! Today was Mother's Day. It was the first one in several years I haven't been filled with resentment. This time last year, I was upset to awaken and find the IUI didn't work. Today, I awoke knowing it surely would only be a matter of days before I was cuddling with you.

The past two weeks have been rough. It's getting warm. I'm swollen, move so slowly, and have a stretch mark that literally grows with every hiccup you have. I have almost grown out of every piece of clothing I own. Maybe that is because I only want to eat sweets.

I do know though to cherish these moments. I will only look back on this pregnancy with the fondest of memories - except for the smell of

159

barbeque and hot sauce!

Your grandpa was moved to a nursing home this week. It has broken my heart to watch him suffer. How I wish you could have been born a month earlier, so he would have the strength to hold you. Always remember that God's timing is better than ours.

As I feel your sweet, little fast kick against me, I have to wonder if you and your grandpa's spirits aren't with each other right now. Maybe you're not ready to come, because you are comforting him. He's very confused with all of the medicines he is on, but he keeps talking about a baby in his room.

He was so, so happy to hear your middle name was going to be "Beatrice," and he loves the name "Olivia" too. I'm sorry you won't grow up having him, but I know he will be watching over you.

I am ready to meet you and am excited for the peace and happiness I know you'll bring this family.

Love,
Mommy

To increase the frustration of not having the baby early – or at least on my due date, literally every single woman I knew who was pregnant that spring had gone early. So what do I do when tears have been cried and nothing has been resolved? I sleep, read, shop and eat – which I did in that order.

I laid in bed for two days and slept and read two books. Oh how I wish I had known how precious, very precious sleep would become. I would have taken more naps and felt less guilty about it when I was pregnant. No, actually, less guilty isn't the way to put it. I wouldn't have given a damn if I had taken a 3 hr nap twice a day, every day. Soak in every ounce of sleep you can from the time you start trying to conceive until the time you have that baby, because as cute as babies are, they are thieves of sleep. Truth.

After two days, I didn't want to risk bed sores (please note the sarcasm), so I felt compelled to move on to my other two comforts of shopping and eating.

The shopping was uneventful, just a

nursing bra (that would later snap under the pressure of my bagoonzas) and jars for homemade baby food. The dinner though was delicious. Shout out to The Old Spaghetti Factory where it is cheap with unlimited bread and dessert is included! It was just what a pregger woman needs.

That night, I laid on the couch and tried to decide why I was extra uncomfortable. Was it the insane amount I had eaten? Gas? By 11:10, I had determined it was not just a new discomfort but instead back contractions.

I sent a text to my sister-in-law that contractions had begun and decided I would do my best to get some sleep.

Tick, Tock. Tick, Tock.
Chapter 25

Back contractions went from ten minutes apart at 11pm on Wednesday night, to eight minutes apart by 2am Thursday morning. However, by 4am, the contractions were only sporadic.

DH and I decided to go to the midwife at 9:30 am, because once again, I thought my water had broken. At least this time, I was having contractions. However once again, the midwife told me that I had just been peeing my pants. I was now at least three now centimeters dilated. In hindsight, I think I should have been given a little credit that perhaps my water was leaking or something!

DH thought I was totally crazy and just peeing my pants to pass time. So off he went to work. During the day there was back pain, lots of cramping and an occasional contraction. I tried cat naps but with little success. I called my mother and told her that I was willing to have the baby on the side of the road in order to walk to get a Sprite and some pretzels from the corner gas station. What a site I'm sure I was to that teenage cashier as I waddled in, wearing my glasses, DH's clothing, and having contractions all to get a snack.

Around 9pm, I called DH at work and told him it was time to come home. Surely this couldn't last much longer. Surely.

By 4am, I awoke with contractions too strong to even think of sleeping. Trying to let DH continue to sleep after working a long day, I put on my headphones and began listening to my hypnobirthing CD.

WHAM! BAM! MY BABY'S KICK JUST BROKE THE DAM! Right where her foot always jabbed into my rib, there was a kick, a pop, and out came the water.

I had tested positive for the Strep B bacteria, so we had been instructed to get to the hospital as soon as my water broke to receive antibiotics. I took a speedy shower, packed the last few things, and woke up DH.

DH groggily awoke and checked the bed sheets upon being told that my water broke. When he didn't see a wet mark, he started to roll over to go back to sleep. In his defense, there had been some water-breaking-false-alarms. Still, I had been in labor over 24 hours at this point. It was time!

By 5:30am we were at the hospital. The nurses hooked me up to the IV. With all the fertility treatments, prenatal appointments, gestational diabetes testing and retesting, I thought I had conquered my fear of needles. My mind may have, but my body had not. I started to pass out at the IV, and the baby's heart rate did a "dippy-do." I don't know what a "dippy-do" is, other than a terrifying moment where they couldn't find her heart rate.

Once things had settled down, I realized I was lying on a mattress that might have well have been plywood. It was so uncomfortable, but we had been instructed in our birth classes to move during labor, so on my feet I went. I swayed. I bounced on a birthing ball. I was on all fours (not even caring for once about the germs on the hospital floor). I moved as much as a 41-week pregnant woman could. Steady contractions continued, but I was only six-centimeters dilated by noon.

The midwife was concerned that at this point I'd been in labor 36 hours and was only six-centimeters dilated. DH was concerned that I'd only packed him a granola bar to eat. Oy

Vey!

So I cranked up my efforts. The midwife had me doing nipple stimulation to induce more contractions. In case you want to clarify what exactly nipple stimulation entails, it's me pinching my freaking nips, while DH tries to be helpful and lend a hand. I know, I'm amazed he's still alive too.

I tried the nipple stimulation. I tried a hot shower. I tried letting DH dance with me (dumbass suggestion from birth class). I even tried smiling at the midwife when she came in. That move really bit me in the ass. She responded to my smile with, "If you're feeling good enough to smile, the labor must not be progressing as well as I'd like it."

Eventually, Pitocin was needed. Around 4 pm, the nurse started the Pitocin, and I had to retreat into my own little world. I was so tired and just could not handle any stimuli. The aromatherapy oils didn't matter anymore and words of encouragement were no longer encouraging. DH had to turn off his NCIS episode on someone with Prader Willy Syndrome (forever grossed out). The hospital phone also had to be ripped from the wall to cease the relative who was incessantly calling. It was just me and the toilet. Yes, me and the toilet.

As the clock ticked on, I found myself stuck on the toilet. Labor is supposed to go more smoothly when your bladder is emptied. Sitting on the toilet during labor is also supposed to subliminally encourage your body to release. What I wasn't warned is that once I sat down on the toilet, there would be no wanting to get up.

Somehow, I did end up back in the bed. Again, on all fours, this time with the midwife's hand up me to check dilation. Don't shove stuff up what's trying to come out. That was easily one of the most painful moments of all of labor. That was also the moment that I decided I wanted Stadol, a drug to help calm me. It was after 7pm. I had been in labor over 44 hours.

Missed Conception

Welcome to the World
Chapter 27

8:48pm. It was time. On my knees, I began to push while hugging the back of the bed. I was so tired, I just so clearly remember the need for the bed to hold me up. The midwife wanted me to turn around though so she could better assist. Once on my back, a surge of strength came over me, and it was time.

I held my legs, curled my body, and I pushed with every ounce of my being. I pushed until I had burst every capillary in my face. Then I pushed more. Most of the time, I waited for the help of a contraction, but sometimes I just kept pushing.

I had waited 48 hours. I had waited for 9 months. I had waited for as long as I could remember, and I was not going to wait any longer.

When it was time to push, I grabbed my ankles and pushed, often not even waiting for a contraction to help me. After hours of support and giving me ice chips, Daddy now sat frozen in a chair by my head. The midwife announced, "Her hair is born."

Daddy reminded me later my response was, "PULL HER OUT BY IT!"

I remember feeling like I was having a bowel movement, but the nurses kept saying what I felt was you. Oops! I began to even laugh during pushing, because a friend had told me it would be like taking the biggest poop of my life! I remember intense short breaths, but not the "ring of fire."

Then the midwife asked if I wanted to pull you out. I reached down, felt your little shoulders, and pulled you on to me as the nurses took off my gown, so you would instantly be skin-to-skin with me.

It was over. You were here.

I felt myself sink back into the

bed and you melt in to me. Daddy gasped to catch his breath with the best smile I have ever seen on his face. We were a family of three!

You were pink and round. You made little gasps for air as your lungs learned to work, and you instinctively knew to search for your first meal. Then Daddy cut the cord, and you became your own, separate little being.

Welcome to the world, Olivia Beatrice. 8lbs, 5oz. 21.5" long. 11:14pm.

Missed Conception

Life Goes On
Chapter 28

Excited to let my mom know Olivia had finally arrived, I had DH hand me my phone as soon as the staff left the room. On my phone was a text from a friend saying something about what a day of extreme grief and joy I was having. Grief?

As soon as I had Olivia on my chest, I had proudly told the nurses and midwife how sweet it was that my dad had been able to hold on, that I had given birth in time. The call made in the labor room to my mom confirmed the contrary. I had not given birth in time. I had been less than four hours too late.

As Olivia was saying hello to the world, my dad had said goodbye. With almost the same timeline of the day as I labored in birth, he had been laboring in death.

I took in the realization that I had just

experienced my greatest loss in life as well as my greatest gain. Only after giving birth, did I realize how the crazy strong pride and intense love I felt for my daughter was the same as that my dad must had felt for me.

As I stared at my beautiful baby, DH and I noticed how her eyes had been swollen to the point of being almond shaped from being in the birth canal so long. My dad had been right, not only had she needed a few extra days, she did look a little Chinese.

As I left the hospital a day and a half later, it was impossible not to collapse in tears. Tears of pure joy. Olivia was all mine, and life had just begun. Not just for her, but for me as well.

We will live happily ever after. Maybe not my vision of what that used to be, but instead, an in-the-moment, I'm staring at my daughter, things will always be okay, kind of happily ever after.

missedconception@aol.com

www.ingramcontent.com/pod-product-compliance
Lightning Source LLC
Chambersburg PA
CBHW060148300526
45790CB00014B/230